FAITH
in the
FACE
of
COVID-19

A SURVIVOR'S TALE

CHRISTINA RAY STANTON

Virginia,
So glad we
survived!
Thank God
Christia
Stanton

LOVING ALL NATIONS PRESS
NEW YORK, NEW YORK

For permission requests, write to the publisher at the address below:

Loving All Nations Press
150 Nassau Street, 4G
New York City, NY 10038
christinarstanton@gmail.com
christinaraystanton.com

Ordering Information:
Special discounts are available on quantity purchases by corporations, associations, and others. For details, contact the publisher at the address above.

Project Manager: Marla Markman, MarlaMarkman.com
Editor: Tammy Ditmore, Editmore.com
Cover and Book Design: Kelly Cleary, kellymaureencleary@gmail.com

Publisher's Cataloging-in-Publication Data

Names: Stanton, Christina Ray, author.

Title: Faith in the face of COVID-19 : a survivor's tale / Christina Ray Stanton.

Description: New York, NY: Loving All Nations Press, 2020.

Identifiers: LCCN: 2020916309 I ISBN: 978-1-7337452-3-9 (pbk.) I 978-1-7337452-4-6 (ebook) I 978-1-7337452-5-3 (audio)

Subjects: LCSH Stanton, Christina Ray. I COVID-19 (Disease) I Healing--Religious aspects--Christianity. I Christian life. I Spiritual healing. I BISAC BIOGRAPHY & AUTOBIOGRAPHY / Personal Memoir I BIOGRAPHY & AUTOBIOGRAPHY / Religious

Classification: LCC BT732.5 .S735 2020 I DDC 234/.131--dc23

978-1-7337452-3-9 (Softcover)
978-1-7337452-4-6 (eReaders)
978-1-7337452-5-3 (Audiobook)

Library of Congress Control Number: 2020916309

Printed in the United States of America

Dedication

I would like to thank Sarah Anderson for inspiring me to write this book, and for her ongoing friendship and support.

I would like to thank my husband for helping to keep me alive during COVID. He is my Rock during times of tumult and in times of calm.

I would like to thank everyone who sent me words of encouragement and who prayed for me while I was sick—I believe it all kept me here on this earth a little while longer.

Proceeds from this book will benefit
Loving All Nations (lovingallnations.org),
which seeks to help the poor, vulnerable, and
marginalized of the world.

For more information about this book, visit
www.christinaraystanton.com

TABLE *of* CONTENTS

1 WAVING...1
Sunday, March 22

2 **To Host or Not to Host**...................7
Monday, March 2

3 A TRIP TO THE HOSPITAL.............11
Sunday, March 22, Morning

4 9/11 LUNGS..............................21
Sunday, March 22, Afternoon

5 **A Day in My Previously Normal Life**...........27
Friday, March 13

6 SOME BAD NEWS........................37
Sunday, March 22, Evening

7 DISTRACTIONS vs. PRAYER..........43
Sunday, March 22, Night

8 **Due to the Coronavirus...**.............49
Saturday, March 14

9 NOTHING MORE WE CAN DO
FOR YOU................................59
Monday, March 23, Morning

10 GROCERIES AND MESSAGES
AND PRAYERS..........................67
Monday, March 23, Afternoon

11 IT'S TRYING TO KILL ME.............75
Monday, March 23, Evening

12 Shutting Down Around Us 85
Monday, March 16, Morning

13 ABOUT LAST NIGHT 97
Tuesday, March 24, Morning

14 Looking for a Test 107
Monday, March 16, Evening

15 GOING DOWNHILL 113
Wednesday, March 25, Afternoon

16 Something Is Wrong 121
Tuesday, March 17

17 HOSPITAL, TAKE #2 131
Wednesday, March 25, Evening

18 Isolated on My "Mini-Vacation" 141
Friday, March 20

19 FIFTY/FIFTY 151
Wednesday, March 25, Night

20 BACK HOME AGAIN 159
Thursday, March 26

21 ROAD TO RECOVERY 171
Tuesday, March 31; Thursday, April 2

22 NEW-BIRTH DAYS 177
Friday, April 3; Sunday, April 5

23 RESURRECTED 181
April 12, Easter Sunday

24 EPILOGUE 187

"My mind and my body may grow weak, but God is my strength; he is all I ever need." Psalm 73:26

1
WAVING
Sunday, March 22

I bet I'll be able to breathe easier if I'm lying on my side.

Slowly and deliberately, I shifted to my left. Brian was awake instantly, propping himself up on his pillow so he could see me. "Are you okay?"

Even though he was trying to be comforting, my husband could not disguise the anxiety in his voice. Wanting to reassure him—and myself—I answered, "I'm fine. If I'm lying down, I'm fine."

He sank back onto the bed beside me. Now that I was on my side, I was staring straight at the bucket on the floor between the bed and the sofa.

Oh man, I have to go AGAIN.

The bucket had been placed in the bedroom when I could no longer walk the few steps to the bathroom just outside the door. Slowly, I hoisted myself up to a seated position, then mustered all my strength to make it to the bucket just in time. I sat for several minutes, trying to gather the resolve for my next move.

Finally, I rose and stumbled a few feet to the sofa, where Brian had set up a nest of necessities Wednesday, when I felt so bad that I retreated to the guest bedroom to isolate myself from Brian's brother and his two daughters. The supplies included Gatorade, gallon jugs of water, towels for when I threw up, Tylenol, a thermometer. He had also left an array of food there, but it was untouched—I had lost my desire for food when I lost the ability to taste it. I stretched out on the sofa and began my daily "job": drinking as much fluid as I could get down.

"Do you think you have a temperature?" Brian asked. He had joined me in this makeshift "isolation ward" the day before, when he started experiencing some weird symptoms and decided to retreat in hopes of sparing the rest of the family.

"I don't think so." I spoke in short bursts, trying to conserve my breath. "It comes in waves ... I read an article ... about COVID ... talked about 'waving' ... a new term ... maybe that's what I'm doing."

"Well, we don't know if you have COVID," Brian said, dismissing my theory. "Christina, why don't you stand up and move a little bit? You've been lying around for days."

I stood up and began shuffling toward the other side of the small room. The room started spinning and my vision dimmed suddenly, as if I had entered a tunnel.

I'm about to faint!

I flung myself on the bed, my face bathed in sweat.

Brian was fully awake now, standing over me, eyes wide. "You can't even walk across the room?" He could not hide the fear on his face.

I faced my own feelings of fear and dread as the room slowly stopped spinning.

"Brian, I hear ... when trouble breathing ... it's time to go to the hospital. Maybe ... that's what this is. Time to go?"

Brian hesitated, then conceded, "Yeah, maybe so. I mean, if

you can't even get out of the bed anymore because you might faint ..."

I was both reassured and unnerved that he had agreed with me.

The hospital. Wow. It's gotten to this so quickly. The only time I've ever been to the hospital was when I was twelve and got my appendix out. I made it all the way to fifty before I thought about going again. Guess my lucky streak has ended?

Ever the planner, I began ticking off what I thought I'd need at the hospital. "Brian, can you ... get my backpack ... my computer and cell ... chargers, my wallet ... ID in wallet? Water."

Brian began gathering items from around the room and making his own list. "I'll bring the masks and the gloves."

"Brian, what hospital are we going to?" I suddenly realized that I didn't know anything about medical care in Tampa, and we were reluctant to wake Brian's brother to ask his advice.

Brian sat heavily on the bed, momentarily stumped. "Let me Google it," he proposed, pulling out his phone. After a few minutes, he said, "It looks like Hillsborough Hospital[1] is the place to go around here. I see here that they've set up a COVID-19 triage. Let's go with that."

"OK," I rasped. "But how are we gonna get there?"

"Riiiiight," said Brian, thinking aloud. "My brother picked us up from the airport. And whatever you have, whether it's COVID or not, you're probably contagious." Staring straight ahead, Brian continued to tick off our options. "Yeah, that's a dilemma. We can't use Lyft or Uber."

"Don't call 9-1-1," I said. "Might take forever to get

---

1 Not the real hospital name.

here—we're out in the boonies." I feared my resolve might waver if I had to wait a long time for an ambulance.

"We'll just have to use my brother's car," Brian said finally. "We really don't have any other great options. I'm going to call Sean," he said, reaching for his phone to call his brother, who was on the floor below.

I looked down at my clothes—leggings and a t-shirt.

Man, I haven't taken a shower since Friday morning. I feel so gross when I go a day without washing myself! But I don't have the energy to change clothes or clean up.

I rose slowly and walked toward the bedroom door as Brian began talking to his brother.

"Sean, I need to get Christina to the hospital. Can we please use your car? Great, thanks. Get yourself and the girls to a room and close the door. We're going to come down now."

Brian grabbed my backpack, opened the bedroom door, and headed down the stairs, shouting, "I'm going to get the car out of the garage and drive it up to the front door to save you some steps."

As I reached the bedroom door, I noticed my black winter coat hanging on a hook. I hadn't touched it since we arrived from New York five days earlier.

I'm going to take this with me, just in case I get chills in the car. Who knew I'd need a winter coat in Florida in March?!

I crept forward, leaving the bedroom area for the first time since I had walled myself in on Wednesday, but froze at the top of the stairs.

No way I can walk down these stairs. Holding on to the rail won't help me if I faint.

Slowly, I sat down on the carpet, swung my legs over the

first step, and perched on the edge. Putting my weight on my hands, I slowly lowered myself down, one step at a time.

Don't forget to breathe. Take deep breaths ...

I was concentrating fully on each step when I suddenly heard Sean calling out from his bedroom at the bottom of the stairs. "Are you out yet?"

"No," I said, as loudly as I could. "Need more time!" I had to stop again to rest.

Look at all this drama I'm causing his family! I certainly do NOT want my nieces watching me scooting down the stairs. They might freak out. They've certainly never seen Aunt Christina like this before.

The staircase ended at the kitchen. Carpet turned into tile, which was harder to crawl across, especially since I was dragging my coat. I was so grateful to see Brian come through the front door. He helped me off the floor, and I clutched his arm, balancing myself as we shuffled down the hall and out the door. I blinked as my eyes adjusted to the brilliant sunshine.

Man, what gorgeous weather. Such a contrast to the gloomy, rainy, and cold New York winter we left behind on Tuesday. I can't believe it's this sunny and I can't believe I feel this bad.

As I climbed into the car, I suddenly had a flash of how drastically my life had changed in just a few short weeks. In fact, it seemed like the whole world had changed in less than a month.

2

To Host
or Not To Host

Monday, March 2

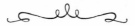

"I t's Here," read the headline on the cover of the *New York Post*.

"Brian, did you see this?" My husband was getting dressed for work in the bedroom as I thumbed through the newspaper in the living room. I didn't have to raise my voice much to be heard across our small apartment. "They have verified that someone in New York City has tested positive for the coronavirus. It's a 39-year-old Manhattan woman who caught the virus while visiting Iran with her husband. According to this article, they both seem okay and are recovering. They're contacting everyone on the flight.

"And another person died from the virus yesterday in the Seattle area. That makes two people who have died from the virus there in just a few days."

"Oh, wow," Brian answered from the bedroom, sounding concerned.

But I was reassured when I saw an article about New York's effort to fight this new virus. "I would like to get a goal of 1,000 tests per day capacity within one week because the more testing, the better," Governor Andrew Cuomo said. "Once you can test a person that's positive, then you can isolate that person so they don't infect other people."

This is awesome—they're clearly on top of it. Testing and isolating will stop this virus in its tracks. Just like they did when that Doctors Without Borders volunteer brought Ebola back here a few years ago. He was quarantined immediately, and it stopped the spread of Ebola in New York City before it started. That's all we need to do again! Geez, I haven't thought about that doctor in a while. I hope he's doing well. God bless him!

"Christina, when are the girls getting here?" Brian asked as he walked to the kitchen and opened the fridge.

"Hmmm, dunno. Maybe around the twelfth or thirteenth? I'll check," I said, as I began searching for my dog-eared black pleather-bound calendar.

I know I'm an old-school dinosaur with this thing. Everyone puts their appointments in their phones or online nowadays—but some things die hard.

Locating my calendar underneath some stray sections of the *Post*, I flipped to the month of March. "Looks like they fly in from Tampa on Saturday, March 14, at 11:40 a.m. They are flying in and out of Newark. I can pick them up, but can you take them back to Newark when they leave the next Wednesday? I start a five-day tour that day."

"Christina, I have to be at work then, too. You know that. Are you going to be free the other days they're here? You haven't had four days off in a row in years. You know *I* won't have any days off when they are here."

"Well," I began, my voice climbing a few pitches, "I have a few short three-hour tours here and there, but I figured they could walk around on their own then, or hang with you for a few hours at your office, or they can go on the tours with me. I mean, I've been a licensed New York City tour guide for twenty-five years. If you're looking for an aunt to explore the city with—these girls have hit the jackpot!"

Brian was skeptical. "Do you *really* think they'll like your Tribeca architecture and Wall Street history tours? They're in that specialized, difficult International Baccalaureate program in high school and probably need an academic break—they'll be on *vacation*. They probably just want to have fun and go shopping!"

His frustration was mounting. "Christina, why did you offer to bring them up here for their spring break if you don't actually have the time to spend with them?"

Indignant, I defended myself. "Because, Brian, I love them so much and wanted to do something special for them. It's a big year for them. It's been tough since their mom got deployed overseas, and Janelle is graduating from high school in May. I thought a trip to New York City would make a great graduation gift. Hey, it's every kid's dream to come play in New York City—and they'll have fun whether I'm busy or not! I'm sure it will work out."

"That's great and all," Brian admonished, "but when you want to do something nice for someone, make sure you have the time to actually do it."

He kissed me on the head, grabbed his backpack, and headed out for work, leaving me frustrated and sheepish. "I'm doing the best I can," I said to the empty room.

I picked up my calendar and studied the remaining twenty-nine days of March. I flipped the page to April. Then to May. As I looked through the big boxes representing the days of 2020, I felt a knot growing in my stomach. I couldn't find a single blank date. Marriott work hours were scribbled into each week; lines with arrows at each end signaled the beginning and end of multi-day tours with a student tour company; evenings were blacked out for the short-term mission trip events I would host. Not written in the calendar—yet—were the hours I would devote to my nonprofit organization or last-minute tours for private clients or the days I would run to Florida to visit my mom or the weeks I would lead mission trips to South Africa or Madagascar. And what about my book talks? In the ten months since my book *Out of the Shadow of 9/11* had been published, I had been invited to speak at multiple churches and schools and book clubs, and the invitations were still coming. I love sharing my testimony about how God used our terrifying 9/11 experiences to change our lives, so how could I turn down those requests? But then, I love *everything* I'm involved in—how can I turn *anything* down?

I stared at the ceiling and shook my head.

It's the beginning of March, and I pretty much know what I'll be doing every day for the rest of the year. This schedule looks worse than last year—and I thought last year was awful. This is completely unsustainable. How do I get out of this? How did I get INTO this?

I set the calendar on my lap and sank into the couch. Closing my eyes, I groaned and voiced a quick prayer: "Lord, please help me get through another grueling year."

3
A TRIP TO THE HOSPITAL

Sunday, March 22, Morning

A s soon as I settled into the car, tears began rolling down my cheeks. I tried to brush them away quickly, hoping this didn't signal another crying jag. I had spent four hours sobbing on the sofa the day before, which was not at all like me.

Brian, who had also cried several times in the past few days, began praying out loud, "Lord, please help Christina. Please heal her, please give wisdom to the doctors at the hospital who will work on her." He flipped on a Christian radio station and praise songs filled the car. "How Great Is Our God" was interrupted by occasional directions from the GPS. "IN ONE HUNDRED FEET, TURN RIGHT ONTO SOUTH FALKENBURG ROAD."

I tried to distract myself by staring out the window. We had left Sean's lush suburban neighborhood behind and were traveling through mile after mile of random shopping centers, car dealerships, fast-food chains, and billboards.

Emperor's Gentlemen's Club, Deja Vu Showgirls ... dang, there are a lot of strip clubs here. Where is "here" anyway? I don't even know what town this is! Just can't believe it's come to this—on my way to some random hospital. This is nuts.

My eyes were burning, my face felt flushed and hot, my

body ached, my throat hurt, my breathing was shallow; the forty-minute drive seemed endless. It was almost 9 a.m. when we drove over a bridge and up a ramp and stopped the car outside the emergency room. We pulled in behind two cars near the curb. Hospital employees wearing several layers of scrubs and masks congregated near the passenger windows, talking to the vehicle occupants.

We've arrived, but it's time to buckle up. I think I'm in for a rocky ride.

Brian pulled over and said, "I'm glad I packed the masks because I saw on the hospital's website that they are requiring patients who come to the emergency room to wear one." He pulled two masks out of my backpack and handed one to me.

I slipped it over my ears, making sure it covered my mouth and nose. A young woman encased in multiple layers of scrubs approached my side of the car, tapped on the window, and pointed down with her finger. Brian leaned over me and pushed the button to lower my window. "Hey, we think we have the virus and we need help," he yelled. "My wife can't breathe."

The young woman retreated a step. After a moment, she asked, "Can she walk?"

I lacked the breath to make myself heard through the mask, and I was crying too hard to talk anyway. But watching Brian and the nurse talking over me just made me cry even harder. The young woman retrieved a wheelchair, and I slowly opened the car door.

"I'm going to try to get tested for COVID while I'm here, so I'll park the car and meet you inside," Brian instructed. I nodded my reply as I transitioned carefully from the car to the wheelchair. The young woman was being careful not to touch me as I balanced my backpack, bottle of Gatorade, and coat on my lap. She whisked me into the hospital and through a series of corridors that appeared to be employee-only areas. We passed one person shrouded like my wheelchair pusher and then another wearing normal scrubs. When we passed someone wearing simple scrubs but no mask, I quickly tilted my head down. I was worried about being contagious but also embarrassed by my tears.

I'm fifty years old! Why can't I control my crying? I need to put my big-girl panties on!

The young woman wheeled me into a small room that looked like an office, with a window into the hallway. A man stepped into the room, wearing extra layers of scrubs, a mask, and a full-face transparent visor. His eyes were the only part of his body that I could see.

"Hello, I'm Jared. I'm the nurse who will be taking care of you. What's your name, where are you from, and why are you here?" He was pleasant and professional but wasted no time. My throat was tight and raspy through the tears, and I struggled to speak loud enough to project through the mask.

"I'm pretty sure I caught COVID ... I feel so bad ... have never felt like this before. Every time I stand ... feel like fainting. Must be breathing issues. That's why I came here. My husband and I just got to Tampa ... five days ago. Last Tuesday. We're from New York City."

"Oh, you're from New York?" His tone changed as he lowered his clipboard to look me straight in the eye. "How'd you end up down here?" he asked, his eyes narrowing.

I struggled to answer his question—it was such a long story, and I didn't have the breath to explain it all. I wasn't sure why it would matter. I had heard that New Yorkers might soon be quarantined if they tried to leave the city; cases were spiking quickly there, and no one else in the country wanted to open the door to New Yorkers carrying COVID.

I hope he doesn't think I traveled recklessly in order to get here!

I caught a glimpse of Brian passing by the room's long rectangular window and raised my arm to wave at him. But I quickly put my hand back down, sensing Jared's disapproval.

Abruptly, Jared placed a hospital tag on my wrist, then stepped behind the wheelchair and rolled me down a hall for several feet. He backed me into another room.

Oh, look, this one has a bed! I guess that means I'm officially admitted? Does the switcheroo mean something?

As I slowly transitioned from the wheelchair to the hospital bed, Jared said, "I'm going to take your temperature and blood samples and measure your blood oxygen level, but first I'll give you a shot so your blood won't clot. When you're in bed and not moving around like usual, you can get blood clots." He put a needle into my belly while saying, "You'll feel a sharp burning sensation."

Dang, he wasn't kidding about that. He's worried about me getting blood clots? Does he think I'm going to be here in bed for that long?

While he conducted the other tests, I studied the room, which was roughly 300 square feet. My bed was the only one in the room, and there was a toilet and sink near the foot of the bed, not in a separate space. A lace curtain covered the small rectangular window positioned high over my head, while a small TV hung from the ceiling. To the left of the toilet was a glass door, which led into a small anteroom between my room and the hallway.

"We're going to give you a chest X-ray, okay? Just lie still," Jared said. A person with a ponytail entered the room—I wasn't initially sure if it was a man or a woman under all the protective layers—pushing a big contraption. My chest was X-rayed quickly, then the employee rolled the contraption out into the anteroom and closed the door to my room tightly. I watched her (it was a woman) take off her gloves and throw them into a bin. She pressed a button on a mounted hand sanitizer dispenser and rubbed the liquid thoroughly on her hands several times. Only after she had shed her extra layers and washed her hands did she move into the hallway. I was beginning to understand that I was in a specialized quarantine room.

Jared announced, "Okay, we're going to measure your blood pressure."

"Need to tell you," I said, wheezing, "I have abnormally low blood pressure. Have all my life."

"Good to know," Jared replied nonchalantly. "Okay, I need you to stand up and sit down quickly, then stand up again and remain standing until I tell you to sit down."

Although tethered to several cords, I stood up and sat down quickly while Jared monitored a device.

"Okay, now stand up and stay standing."

I stood up. After a few seconds, I said, "I gotta sit down now. Think I'm gonna faint."

"Just a little bit longer," Jared commanded.

C'mon, girl, you can do it!

"Okay, you can sit." Jared was still watching the monitor.

I collapsed back into bed triumphantly, feeling like I had just crossed the finish line of a marathon.

"Wow, you weren't kidding—you really do have low blood pressure. And your pressure drops dramatically when you sit back down. We have to get that stabilized. What you thought were breathing issues was really probably just your low blood pressure acting up."

"I see," I said, wishing Brian were with me to hear his analysis. I ventured, "My husband is here. If we both get admitted, can we stay in this same room?"

"No, people in quarantine have to stay alone," Jared replied matter-of-factly, not even looking at me. Without missing a beat, he reported, "Your temperature is 101. For sure you need an IV."

My tears were still flowing—although they had slowed to a trickle—when he put a needle in my right arm and hooked me up to an IV. As soon as the drip began, my tears stopped. I was amazed. It was almost as if the liquid from the IV had a direct effect on the liquid coming out of my eyes! Maybe I had been crying because I was dehydrated?

Wow, I feel instantly more comfortable. So much better. Praise the Lord!

"This next test will be the last one for now," Jared told me. "I'll give you some time to rest after this." He reached behind him and picked up a swab on a long wooden stick. "This is the COVID test. This will hurt a little," he said, shoving the swab far, far up my nose. I clenched my hands into fists to keep from jerking away. He reached for another long swab and stuck it in my mouth toward the back of my throat. I gagged.

"The wait for the results has been reduced recently for this test, which is great! It used to take eight hours or more, but you should know in about five hours," Jared said genially. "If you need anything, press the button, and a nurse will bring it to you. However, we have a lot of personal protective equipment to take on and off, so try to bring someone in only if you *really* need assistance."

"Thank you," I said, relieved I could rest after the barrage of tests.

Jared walked to the other side of the room and stripped off his visor, mask, and gloves, dropping them into the trash can. He then proceeded to the sink, where he wet his hands, then turned off the faucet while he got soap out of the dispenser. He rubbed his hands together several times to create a thick lather, then scrubbed the back of his hands, between his fingers, and under his nails. He rubbed and rubbed for at least a minute and then rinsed his hands thoroughly. He then walked into the anteroom and sanitized his hands as I had seen the X-ray technician do.

I have never in my life seen someone wash their hands like that! Is that how we're actually supposed to wash our hands? What a production! I must be so, so contagious. My body is like a lethal weapon. I'm a danger to others! What an awful thought.

My phone buzzed, and I grabbed it from the table beside me. "Brian, are you still here? What's happening to you?" I was surprised I could speak without being winded. It had to be the IV.

"Well, they wouldn't give me a test because I don't meet all the criteria for the coronavirus," Brian said. "My temperature was normal, I don't have a cough, my throat's only a little sore. I'm not experiencing all the symptoms."

"B-b-but," I protested, "did you tell them you're from New York? That we just came from there? That I might be COVID-positive? Your digestive system hasn't been normal, you *have* had a temperature in the last few days." The more I talked, the angrier I got.

"I can't *believe* they wouldn't give you a test—you should have *made* them! Whatever I have, you have it too, and you might get it as bad as me—it just hasn't hit you yet."

"I know, Christina." Brian tried to calm me. "Just concentrate on *you* feeling better. Are you going to come home now? Have they told you if they're keeping you?"

I stopped, realizing I had not asked and Jared had not given me any idea of what was in store for me next. "I really wasn't told about any particular treatment plan. But I know my blood pressure needs to be stabilized and I have to wait for the COVID test results."

"Then there's nothing for me to do other than go back to Sean's house," Brian said reluctantly. "Call me and keep me updated." As I put my phone down on the bed, the hospital phone on the nightstand began ringing. I hesitated, then picked it up. "Hello?"

"It's Patient Check-in. I need to ask you some questions to finish checking you into the hospital."

Wow. They can't do this face to face? I have to do this over the phone because my physical presence is potentially deadly. I guess this is my new normal.

By the time I had answered all the questions, it was noon and I was exhausted.

Well, looks like I'm free to nap as long as I want. It's weird to be alone, though. I'm alone in a random hospital in an area I rarely visit.

18

I'm almost never alone—especially not in March! In March I'm supposed to be touring scores of tourists around New York City. Maybe I'll wake up and it will all be some crazy nightmare.

4
9/11 LUNGS

Sunday, March 22, Afternoon

Instead, I woke about four hours later, shivering and alone in an ice-cold hospital room. I found a thin robe and a thin sheet on the bed and spread both across my body. I spied my black coat splayed across the nightstand and added it to the layers, but my makeshift bedding did not stretch to my bare, cold feet.

The bottle of Gatorade on the bedside table was almost empty, so I propped myself up on the bed and scanned the bare room. No water fountain, no cup, no blanket, nothing to eat. Moving carefully because of my IV, I slid my backpack toward me from the bottom corner of the bed and rifled through it, feeling a surge of joy when my hand fell on a crinkly plastic water bottle.

Woohoo! Man, good thing Brian packed this. After seeing all the hoopla those nurses have to go through, I don't want to bother them just to ask for water and a blanket. Maybe I'll make a list and hit them with it when someone comes in.

I noticed the IV bag was nearly empty and realized the fluids had done their work. I looked at my right arm, which was hooked up to the IV, and then to my left hand, hooked up to a machine to measure my blood pressure, then straight ahead at the toilet in the room, plotting my next move. I threw my legs over the side of the bed, stood up, and tried to drag everything with me, but the blood pressure wire was too short. I picked up the cord box and unhooked it. Free from that machine, I began dragging the IV stand to the toilet, but it got caught on the leg of the bed. I tried jostling it, but gave up after a few minutes.

Hmmm, if I extend my IV'd arm to where the cord is stretched to its full length, my body can hover over the toilet. The cord isn't long enough to allow me to sit on it. Okay, well, this is what I got. I get to be a dude and pee standing up.

After I finished, I was able to grab the empty Gatorade bottle on the nightstand and fill it from the sink. I climbed back in bed and reconnected the blood pressure monitor.

Whoa, look at those elevated numbers. So much higher than before all the toilet activity. Just lie back down on the bed and take deep breaths. If I have a heart attack, will these people come help me? Looks like they're limiting how much they come into my room so they won't get exposed to possible COVID. Do they have a monitor at the nurses' station where they can check on me? Could I die with no one realizing it until they make their next round?

When the numbers descended, I positioned the makeshift covers over me and breathed a sigh of satisfaction.

WHEW! I did it! Without any help from a nurse! Apparently, I'll be fending for myself to a big degree, so I need to get resourceful! Oh no. I need to pee again.

Just then, a tall man stepped into the room. He was covered head to toe, like all the other employees I had encountered here.

"Hello, I'm Dr. Deepali. So, I understand you have just come to Tampa from New York and you think you have COVID?"

"Yes, that's correct," I answered, as he walked to a computer on a stand built into the wall. He began typing away. I propped myself up on the bed and tried to catch a glimpse of what he was writing. Although I could see white letters, I was too far away to isolate words or sentences that could tell me anything about my condition. But I could make out a small bit written in orange at the bottom left corner of the screen: COVID+.

I sank back onto the pillow and wondered whether that little tag signified I had been tested or that I had tested positive for the coronavirus that causes COVID-19.

"So, tell me more." The doctor seemed unaware of my attempts to read the chart.

"I think I caught COVID last week or the week before in New York City, maybe even the day we left, which was last Tuesday. By the way, there's something important I need to let you know. I have '9/11 lungs.'"

"What?" The doctor finally turned from the computer to face me. Even through the mask and visor I could see he was perplexed.

"Yes, I'm one of many people whose health was affected due to the September 11th attacks. I experienced 9/11 firsthand. When the towers came down, I inhaled the toxic dust that has now been linked to sixty different cancers. It's left me with scarred lungs and other health issues, and will probably make whatever I have worse. Just wanted you to know some of my health background."

"Huh." He turned back to the computer. "Thanks for letting me know."

I wasn't surprised that this was the first time the doctor

had heard of 9/11 lungs. I had seen many doctors in New York who weren't aware of it either—even though a lot of us there are suffering from the condition.

I blurted out the question that was bothering me most. "Do you know what my COVID test results are? It's after four o'clock now, and I took the test around eleven. They told me it would take five hours to find out the results."

Still facing away from me, the doctor continued typing. "We don't know yet, and we're still waiting on other test results for you as well. We're going to keep you overnight for observation, mainly due to your blood pressure."

"I see," I said. "You'd probably want to keep me here since I might be COVID-positive too, right?"

"Actually, no," he countered, a little harshly, in my opinion. "We wouldn't necessarily keep you here if you tested positive; that alone won't get you a bed here. Your body has to show distress to continue to stay in the ER. We need our beds for those who are being incapacitated by the virus."

I was silent as the doctor turned back to his computer. But my brain was spinning.

I've never felt this bad before. My body is definitely in distress. Isn't that what a hospital is for? Why is it not for me?

But I didn't ask the doctor any of those questions. I didn't want to be *that* patient. Instead, I said, "Could you ask someone to come in to help me? Since I'm staying, I need a few things, and I haven't eaten yet today."

"Sure," he said. "I'll send someone in. Just rest."

As he exited, he performed the same elaborate shedding of his uniform, hand-washing, and sanitizing as everyone else who had stepped inside my room.

I lay back, exhausted and confused. If I didn't have COVID, why did I feel so bad? And why was everyone treating me like I was toxic?

I thought back to the first day it dawned on me that the pandemic was going to have a big impact on my life. Could that have been only nine days ago?

5

A Day in My Previously Normal Life

Friday, March 13

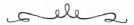

"Brian, I'm running off to the Marriott. I'll clean the apartment and assemble the pullout couch when I get home, okay?" I opened the front door and grabbed the *New York Post* from the carpet in the hall.

"Hey, I'm ready too," Brian called as he rushed toward the door. "We can ride the subway together."

I stopped in the hall, surprised. "I thought you all decided Wednesday that the Redeemer office employees would work remotely from here on out. So, why are you going into the office to work today?"

"We told employees that they could grab what they needed out of their cubicles for the rest of the week, but Monday would be our official closing date. I have a few odds and ends to finish there in order to be ready for Monday."

"Got it!" I nodded as he closed the door behind him.

We veered right out of our apartment building, rapidly covering the few blocks to our closest subway entrance.

"Man, this subway is an obstacle course at 8:30 in the morning," I griped, dreading the six sets of stairs and two trains that lay between us and work.

"Yes, but it sure is quick!" Brian countered. "We can get

from Downtown Manhattan to Midtown in less than a half hour."

"True, true! I just probably need my morning coffee," I conceded, as we shoved our way into a packed train car. We both grabbed a pole to brace ourselves against the bumpy ride.

"Well, maybe if your backpack wasn't so heavy, the trek wouldn't be so arduous," Brian teased.

"I know. I keep hauling around that huge book about Amy Carmichael. I'm fascinated by the mission work she did in India. I've made it about halfway through the book. I never, ever have time to read it, but I keep dragging it around with me because I always think at one point I'll miraculously have the time." I sighed. "It takes me all day just to read through this thing to see what's happening in the world," I said, lifting up the newspaper.

With my free hand, I clumsily opened the *New York Post*, and my eye fell on an alarming headline: "9/11 responders and survivors at risk for contracting coronavirus, officials warn." I quickly scanned the article. "Look at this, Brian," I said, shoving the newspaper to him. "It says people like us who inhaled the deadly toxins during 9/11 might be more susceptible to the coronavirus. It could have a worse effect on us potentially, too, because our lungs have been compromised."

"Oh, wow," he said, scanning the article. "That makes me a bit nervous."

"Me too."

I retrieved the newspaper and continued to thumb through it, mainly just scanning the headlines: "Tonight begins a 30-day travel ban for Americans to/from Europe." "NYC coronavirus count stays at 95, city has no plans to shut down: de

Blasio." I chuckled at New York City Mayor Bill de Blasio's comment, "New Yorkers don't scare easily!"

Heck no, they don't! It would take a LOT more than ninety-five people infected out of almost nine million and only 325 in a state of nineteen million to get New Yorkers to turn on their heels—for anything!

In fact, I had been surprised to see three people wearing masks in the train packed with morning commuters.

Well, maybe those three scare easily. But for all the rest, it's business as usual!

Brian brought me back to reality when he asked, "Do you think the girls are nervous to come up here? Do they know some things are closed?"

"Well, I talked to them last night and told them to have low expectations about what we'll be able to do because of so many closings. They were okay with that. I know your brother doesn't seem worried by the pandemic because he's okay with them coming up. So I guess it's all a go!"

As the train rolled into the 34th Street/Herald Square station, I gave Brian a quick goodbye kiss. "Love you, honey!" I said, darting out of the sliding doors. He had two more stops to ride to get to his office at Redeemer Presbyterian Church. I put my fingers in my ears to block out the sound of jackhammers—the soundtrack to the endless construction in Midtown—and hurried the three blocks up 6th Avenue to the Marriott Vacation Club. Traveling with the tide of people heading my way, I dodged the wave of workers rushing downstream and sidestepped the trash spilling from the always overflowing trash cans around Macy's. Nothing seemed different about today's morning dance—except for a few people wearing masks, who were still rare enough to be very noticeable. I passed the man who begged for money every day as he opened the door for McDonald's customers, turned right onto 37th Street, and entered the Marriott. "Hey, Jocelyn!"

"Hey there—good morning," my boss responded cheerily as I sank into my chair in the compact basement office.

"Anyone sign up for my tours today?" I asked, unlocking my cupboard.

"None for your High Line/Chelsea Market tour, but two people signed up for your 9/11 tour," she said, studying the sign-up sheets. "We're at twenty-five percent capacity. People are starting to get scared to travel here because of the pandemic. They're staying home. In fact, no one has signed up for your Sunday and Monday tours."

"Awww …" I responded, my anxiety growing a little.

After a beat, Jocelyn proposed, "Why don't you take those days off? There will be so few people here I don't foresee needing you for anything."

Elated, I bellowed, "Great! My nieces will be in town and canceling my hours here will free up time to do things with them. Thanks!"

Wow, this is a gift! I can just be totally with the girls now! Thank you, Lord!

"Good," Jocelyn answered, pleased—and a little surprised—by my reaction. "Hey, did I see you limping when you walked in?"

"Girl, two walking tours a day are killing my feet. I don't know what to do about it. And I told you I've got these ulcers on the bottom of my left foot. Turning fifty *stinks*! I swear this city is a young person's game. I could walk for miles when I moved here when I was twenty-three. But lately it's gotten more challenging.

"My body may have changed through the years, but my love for the city hasn't. It'll never get old to me: the history, the architecture, the quaint streets. And I *love* being a tour guide."

"I get ya," Jocelyn said, as she finished paperwork at her desk. "All this walking is both good and bad, but it's what we do for a living, right? It's the price we Florida transplants pay for loving this crazy city and wanting tourists to fall in love with it, too."

She handed me a piece of paper. "And look what I have for you this morning."

I turned the paper lengthwise to read it. "A certificate commemorating my one-year anniversary at the Marriott! Wow, I didn't realize it had been a full year! I'm so glad y'all hired me … taking Marriott Vacation Club owners on walking tours has been one of the most fun jobs I've ever had. Central Park, Little Italy/Chinatown, 9/11 memorial, sample sales in the Garment District … I love taking your peeps to my favorite places."

My cell phone rang. Junior Tours was calling. "Jocelyn, this is the owner of the student tour company I work for. I'm going to take the call—I have a few minutes before my 9/11 tour," I said, stepping out of the office for privacy.

"Hey, Christina, this is Mark."

"Hey, dude, what's up?" I answered, with a familiarity that comes from working with someone for a quarter of a century. But I wasn't expecting what he had to say next.

"I have bad news. Your tour starting next Wednesday has

canceled, and there is the possibility all your tours might cancel for the season."

I was shocked. "But Mark, that's fifteen tours—almost sixty days of work altogether!"

No student tours for the year? I tried to understand how something that had been part of my yearly schedule for almost half my life could vanish so quickly.

"Well, groups are getting scared to travel because of the virus, and since Broadway shows collectively closed yesterday, that's an indicator it's just a bad time to visit the city," he said.

"Yes, but they said on the news that Broadway would only be closed for thirty-two days—clearly just to get over the hump of this thing. It's not like the entire theatre season is shot!"

"*I* know that and *you* know that," Mark said. "But I'm just trying to prepare you for what I'm seeing here."

This pandemic must be really getting bad, or people are getting super paranoid. I'm so sad for all those kids who won't get their New York City adventure this year. I love showing teenagers around the city!

"I guess I get it," I admitted. "The mayor has declared a state of emergency in New York City, and believes the coronavirus tally will jump from the ninety-five it is today to a thousand soon. But he's also noting that the stock market isn't closing, he said he won't shut down city schools, and that New Yorkers don't scare easily."

I kept talking, more to myself than to Mark. "So many mixed messages! I can see why tourists are scared and confused and are trigger-happy to cancel their travel plans. But I can't tell if these closures are preventative measures just for precaution, or if we're preparing for a virus war!"

Jocelyn opened the office door and tugged at my shirt sleeve. "Christina, I think the two people on your tour are upstairs waiting."

"Oh, yes, thanks, Jocelyn," I whispered. "Mark, I have to go. Thanks for calling! Keep me updated."

Grabbing my Marriott flag and my backpack full of 9/11 and World Trade Center pictures, I ran up the spiral staircase leading from the office to the lobby. "Hello, folks!" I approached a couple in their sixties who were standing by the concierge desk.

"Welcome! My name is Christina." I brushed aside the worrying news I had just received and conjured up my most professional "tour guide" demeanor. "Let me tell you a bit of what to expect today. We'll take a forty-minute subway ride to the Cortlandt Street station. It exits into the four-billion-dollar Oculus station house designed by Santiago Calatrava—an incredible thing to see. When we make our way out of that complex, we'll be right at the site. We'll see the 9/11 museum, the Firefighter Memorial, the Anne Frank tree and the Survivor Tree, and a new addition to the sixteen-acre World Trade Center site called Memorial Glade. We'll visit both the North and South Towers, where I'll give you details both about the Twin Towers and about the present-day memorial. The entire tour with travel time takes about three and a half hours. Does that sound okay?"

"Wow, that sounds fantastic, Christina!"

"Great, well, let's start on our way!" As we strolled to the yellow R/W subway line at Herald Square, I told the couple,

"During our subway ride down, I could tell you a personal story of what happened to my husband and I during 9/11, which you might find interesting ..."

I love this tour. I feel such a calling to share with others what happened to Brian and I, and it's so awesome to be able to educate people about the attacks of September 11th. This is actually my twenty-fifth anniversary of showing tourists the World Trade Center site. NYC and I have been down a long, long road together.

Exiting the subway at Cortlandt Street, we stepped into the Westfield Mall. "This is a subterranean mall with 125 great stores, but it's really the artwork covering the mall that's truly unique. Follow me outside and we'll discuss it some more," I said, leading them through the exit facing the 9/11 memorial. This was where I usually started my commentary about the Oculus and the One World building. But today, I was stopped short by the sight of a white chain-link barrier blocking the full perimeter of the 9/11 memorial.

Several people milled around near the rope barrier, walking aimlessly and looking agitated. On the other side of the rope were stern-looking policemen, spaced out about every ten feet, backs to the memorial, facing us.

Surprised, I said, "I was just here yesterday. I don't know what's going on with this rope—there was no heads-up about anything closing today. Let's go over and find out what's happening."

As I approached an officer, the three of us saw a sign mounted on a tripod near the rope: "In accordance with the guidance provided by our state and local governments regarding large public gatherings in response to the COVID-19 pandemic, we are temporarily closed."

"Wow, I had no idea they'd be closing today," I apologized. "It wasn't in the news or anything—it must have been decided today at the last minute."

"Does this mean we go back to the Marriott? That the tour is canceled?" asked the gentleman.

"No—not to worry. There's an overlook to the memorial right there," I said, pointing to Liberty Park, a one-acre elevated public park. "We can get a panoramic view of all the points of interest I mentioned earlier." I set out confidently, trying to hide my continued surprise—and mounting concern.

Wow, things are closing fast, with no warning, no heads-up. And there doesn't seem to be an organized response or cohesive plan to the closings. Havoc seems to be reigning—it's some kind of alternative universe. What's New York without the museums and Broadway? What will that mean for tourists? What will that mean for Janelle and Mae when they visit? And what will that mean for those of us who live here?

6
SOME BAD NEWS
Sunday, March 22, Evening

I was half-asleep when my phone buzzed, but I was thrilled to see my husband's name pop up on the screen.

"Hey, Brian, I just saw the doctor," I began.

"Oh, good." Brian cut me off, anxiously. "Did you get the test results? We've all been on edge over here waiting to hear if you're positive or not."

"No! The doctor said they don't seem to know yet, which I think is weird. I'm really anxious to know the results!"

"I've thought a lot about it, and I think you probably don't have the virus," Brian said, trying to sound positive. "I think you just came down with something. Remember how sick you were last year from the flu? That's probably it."

"I hope you're right, Brian," I said, although I did not share his optimism.

He probably should be preparing himself for the worst. For sure this ain't no flu!

I dozed off again after I hung up with Brian, waking when a nurse in many layers of scrubs and a mask backed into my room, her arms loaded with a large tray. "Hello, here's your dinner: pork chops and green beans. It's a low-sodium meal," she explained.

I had no idea why I would need a low-sodium meal.

"I heard you have some requests," she said. "What do you need?"

I glanced at the clock on the wall: 5:30 p.m. More than an hour since I had asked the doctor to send someone in.

I rattled off my list. "Can someone bring in water, a blanket, and some socks?"

"Oh! You didn't get your 'welcome packet'!" my nurse said cheerily, grabbing the hospital phone. "Hey, is anyone available to bring in a welcome packet?" She put the phone down and walked to the door leading to the anteroom, where someone had entered from the hallway and cracked open the transparent door to my room. A bag passed through the crack, and my nurse made sure she didn't touch the gloved hand on the other side of the door during the pass-off.

She hoisted the bag and announced exuberantly, "Here we are!" before ripping open the plastic. "Here is a blanket, some socks, a washcloth, and a big Hillsborough Hospital water jug." She set each item on the nightstand as she pulled them from the bag.

God bless her—she's trying to be cheery in the midst of these yucky circumstances!

Pulling aside my mass of makeshift covers, she picked up the blanket off the nightstand, unfolded it, and threw it over me. Although it was thin, the blanket was incredibly warm, and I was grateful to be warm at last! I didn't ask about changing into a hospital gown or robe. Surprisingly, no one seemed to notice or care that I was still in my street clothes, and I didn't want to go through the hassle of changing. Especially now that I was as snug as a bug in a rug.

"Listen, ma'am," I pleaded as she began putting the hospital socks on my bare feet. "I really need to know if I'm COVID-positive. I need to let my husband know. And the family he's staying with."

I could see the nurse's eyes widen, even though they were shielded by a plastic visor. She straightened up, standing rigidly at the foot of the bed in silence. A second went by; two seconds; three.

Finally, she blurted out, "You are *quite* positive. I don't know why you weren't told." She picked up my water jug and walked it to the sink.

So I was right about the orange writing on my chart! Why didn't the doctor just tell me?

Tears started falling down my cheeks, and my nose began running.

"Here's your water," the nurse said, a hint of sadness in her voice. She set the jug on the nightstand and rolled it closer to my chest. Turning around, she walked to the trash can and began the exit ritual.

I kept my composure until the door closed behind her but began sobbing as I watched her sanitize her hands in the anteroom. I picked up my phone and called Brian.

"I'm positive," I lamented. "You need to tell Sean and the girls."

"Ohhhhh, shoot," Brian said. He began crying too.

"It looks like I'll be here for a while. Nurse Jared told me that 'quarantined people have to be alone,' and I've heard reports on the news that loved ones can't visit COVID-positive people in the hospital. I've also heard that they can be in the hospital for weeks."

A thought struck me. "Should we call United Airlines to

tell them I was probably COVID-positive during our flight last Tuesday? I mean, when the New York woman tested positive after her flight from Iran a few weeks ago, everyone who was on the plane was contacted. But I don't know if they are still doing that?"

"I'll call United. You think of who you might have been around since last weekend."

When I got off the phone, I listed the name of every person I had spent time with since Saturday, March 14th. As I thought about each day, I felt a growing sense of relief when I realized that I had seen very few people apart from Brian, my nieces, and Sean. And most of those encounters had been outdoors, with the exception of our flight from New York City to Tampa.

Thank goodness our plans got changed so that we couldn't get together with Jenny and Lauren while the girls were in New York City. Thank you, Jesus!

After making my list, I pulled my laptop from my backpack and set it up on my belly, feeling an urgent need to reach beyond this room where I was so alone.

I have got to get people to pray for me and Brian and Janelle and Mae and Sean. I'll write a Facebook post and then send individual emails. This is way important!

Logging on to my Facebook page, I wrote:

Friends, I have some sad news. I have tested positive for the virus and am at Hillsborough Hospital in quarantine for the foreseeable future. I was having trouble breathing, which is what brought me to the hospital earlier today. Brian was not allowed to be tested since he didn't show any symptoms.

He is staying in quarantine at a house east of Tampa. Since I have it, he probably does too, however.

Many of you read my book, and so you'll recall that Brian and I have ongoing health issues due to the toxins we inhaled during and after 9/11. Knowing our health is compromised, we tried to evacuate the city last Tuesday. Apparently, it bit us in the butt just as we were on the way out the door.

Please add me and Brian and Brian's family to your personal prayer list, to your Bible study group's prayer list, and if your church has a prayer list, please add us to that as well.

Geez, I want to tag and mention Sean and the girls more specifically in my post, but I really shouldn't since we are in their community. Their friends and neighbors might become concerned if they knew they were next door to COVID-positive people. I'll include them in the private emails to good friends.

One hour passed, then two, while I sat, pecking at my keyboard. Three hours later, I was still reaching out to friends to ask them to become prayer partners. I was delighted to find email information for Mike Sunker, founder of the Christ Church Christian Care Center orphanage in Johannesburg, South Africa. I had visited Mike and the kids at what we call the 5Cs for the past ten years and knew they were prayer warriors! "Mike, I just tested COVID-positive and am in a hospital. I might end up having a bad case of this. Will you have the staff and kids pray for me and Brian, and family members Sean, Janelle, and Mae? You might remember them—they came with me to visit the children at the 5Cs on a mission trip last year."

I decided to broaden my email requests even further. I had been the director of the short-term missions program at Redeemer Presbyterian in New York City for a decade, so I knew pastors all over the world.

The mission teams and I have been faithfully praying for them for years. They would LOVE to have the opportunity to reciprocate! And maybe they'll mobilize their communities and congregants to pray for us as well! Heck, we could have people ALL OVER the world praying!

After writing about a hundred pastors and ministry leaders, I felt strengthened for a task I had been avoiding: calling my mother in Tallahassee. She had no idea about my current state, and I feared she would be mad at me for not keeping her in the loop.

Mom answered after a few rings. "Hi, Chrissy! I haven't heard from you in over a week. How are things up there in New York? Are you having fun with your nieces?"

"Mom," I began, guiltily. Then I rushed to get it all out at once. "I'm not in New York. I'm actually about four hours from you. I'm sorry I didn't let you know, but I've been sick and I'm in a hospital in Central Florida, and it turns out I'm COVID–positive. But I'll be fine, don't you worry."

Mom waited a beat, obviously trying to take in this overload of information. Finally, she said, "You survived 9/11—you're a fighter. I know you'll triumph over this."

I was so relieved and so grateful. Instead of being mad or upset, Mom had just given me a boost of confidence.

She's right. Surely, I'll make it through this. I've been through worse!

7

DISTRACTIONS
VS.
PRAYER

Sunday, March 22, Night

I decided to turn on the little TV hanging from the ceiling, hoping for some distraction. Flipping through the channels, I stopped when I saw a video of New York Governor Andrew Cuomo announcing that "the New York City region is now an epicenter of the pandemic—accounting for roughly five percent of the world's confirmed cases. Temporary hospitals will be constructed in NYC, and a Navy hospital ship is being deployed to dock in the Hudson and relieve the pressure on overloaded hospitals."

An epicenter? Overloaded hospitals? How did it come to that so quickly?!

I flipped the channel and heard a news anchor report, "Italy has nearly 60,000 confirmed cases and has had more than 5,000 deaths. Seven-hundred-ninety-three succumbed in a single day." I moved quickly away from that channel. But it seemed every TV station was giving coronavirus updates. This was not the distraction I had been hoping for.

I found a rerun of *The Golden Girls* but lost interest quickly. I kept flipping until I finally landed on one of my favorite shows, *Forensic Files*. But I could only stand to watch a few minutes of the show's depictions of death and misery.

I switched off the TV, reached for my laptop, and logged on to the *New York Post*, a newspaper I had read almost every day for twenty-seven years. A featured headline proclaimed, "NYC coronavirus death toll reaches 99." According to the article, 1,800 New Yorkers had been hospitalized, and almost 11,000 had tested positive for the virus. I kept clicking on COVID-related links, reading about the debate over whether to cancel the Tokyo 2020 Olympics, a twelve-year-old girl in Atlanta fighting for her life, and a South African former Olympic swimmer who had just beaten the virus but described it as "by far the worst I've endured." The news was not encouraging.

If a super-fit former Olympian barely survived, and a twelve-year-old child is dying, what could that mean for an overweight, run-down, middle-aged woman like me?! I think it's time to close the Post. *I need something light and fluffy—let me look on Facebook.*

Scrolling through my newsfeed, I tried to skip over the coronavirus articles being shared and reshared by my friends but couldn't avoid them all. I saw headlines about making face masks and overcrowded hospitals and severe coronavirus symptoms in "young Americans."

Ha! According to this article, I'm "young"! It's nice to be called young, but not so nice that thirty-six percent of people between forty-five and sixty-four need to be hospitalized when they catch this virus. And why are people having to make face masks for hospital workers? Why are we so unprepared? Is THIS hospital unprepared too?

Looking for non-COVID news, I discovered a series of posts announcing the death of country singer Kenny Rogers.

Although he had died a couple of days earlier, I had been too sick to notice. His death hit me hard.

I love Kenny! My dad's favorite singer. I grew up with Kenny's music.

"You Decorated My Life" began playing in my mind as my memory filled with thoughts of my dad, who had died of cancer at age of fifty-two, when I was just twenty-three.

It would be so nice to have him around now, but I'm not sure he'd want to be living in this day and age. I'm not sure I do either. I really believed humans had harnessed nature pretty well by this point. I thought pandemics were a thing of the past—that science was advanced enough to nip this kind of stuff in the bud. Has my head been in the clouds? Is this prideful thinking, or am I more ignorant than I thought?

I shut my laptop. I could not take any more news, and I didn't want to read email, look at Facebook, watch TV, or talk to anyone on the phone. I scanned my room, feeling more and more lonely and isolated until my eyes fell on the Bible on the nightstand. I was so grateful now that I had thought to put my Bible in my backpack as we were getting ready to leave the house.

No more attempts at distraction. The only thing I need to be doing is taking my worries to the Lord. It's time to talk to God. I need him desperately right now. Turn to Psalm 116—I love that one. That's a good one for a time like this!

Psalm 116

I love the Lord, because he hears me; he listens to my prayers.

He listens to me every time I call to him.

The danger of death was all around me; the horrors of the grave closed in on me; I was filled with fear and anxiety.

Then I called to the Lord, "I beg you, Lord, save me!"

The Lord is merciful and good; Our God is compassionate.

The Lord protects the helpless; when I was in danger, he saved me.

Be confident, my heart, because the Lord has been good to me.

The Lord saved me from death; he stopped my tears and kept me from defeat.

And so I walk in the presence of the Lord. In the world of the living.

I kept on believing, even when I said, "I am completely crushed," even when I was afraid and said, "No one can be trusted."

What can I offer the Lord for all his goodness to me?

I will bring a wine offering to the Lord, to thank him for saving me.

In the assembly of all his people I will give him what I have promised.

How painful it is to the Lord when one of his people dies!

I am your servant, Lord; I serve you just as my mother did. You have saved me from death.

I will give you a sacrifice of thanksgiving and offer my prayer to you.

In the assembly of all your people, in the sanctuary of your Temple in Jerusalem.

I will give you what I have promised. Praise the Lord!

Tears started rolling down my cheeks again at the beauty of

this psalm and how appropriate it was for this time in my life. It was time to call on the name of the Lord.

Lord, I know you're with me. If it's in your will, please heal me. I'm grateful I was able to get the test to find out I was positive, and thank you for my low blood pressure! It was the tip-off that got me to the hospital ... and got me the test ... and kept me here. Thank you for the care I'm getting at the hospital! Thank you, Lord, for the health of my family. Please guard Brian, Sean, Janelle, and Mae's health! I'm so thankful they're home taking care of each other. Thank you for your Holy Spirit. He's here. And he's got this!

A nurse I hadn't seen before entered the anteroom. "I have two sets of pills for you to take—they're in the small cups on the tray." I picked up each cup and took out the pills.

"What are these?" I asked the nurse, who was covered head to toe. All I could see were her eyes and her ponytail.

"Hydroxychloroquine and Tylenol," she replied.

"Oh, wow," I said enthusiastically. "You all are distributing the medication that's been in the news? I've heard a lot about this medicine—it's supposed to be a miracle worker. I've taken it before, too. Several times when I went on mission trips to countries that have a problem with malaria."

I quickly threw all four pills to the back of my throat and washed them down with a swig from my water jug. "By the way," I said, testing the waters, probing for the information nobody seemed to want to share with me, "am I the only COVID-positive patient here in the hospital?"

"No, we've had others. But honestly, we thought we'd have a lot more by now. We did special training, we opened this wing for patients, all hands are on deck, we have a whole triage with doctors waiting." This nurse seemed eager to chat.

"I mean, this is a big city, a port city. We thought we'd be slammed, and we aren't yet."

"Interesting," I responded. "I don't know the area, but I would have thought there were a lot of cases here, too."

"What?" she asked, seeming surprised. "Are you not from here?"

I shook my head.

"Where are you from, then?"

"New York City," I responded hesitantly, fearing her judgment.

Wow, things are absolutely topsy-turvy right now; I never thought I would ever, ever be embarrassed and ashamed to say I live in New York City.

"Oh, *cool*! I was there last year and had so much fun!" she exclaimed.

Oh, honey, it might have been fun and cool then. But the city is totally NOT fun and cool right now.

As the nurse engaged in her elaborate scrub-down and left my room, I remembered how the city had transformed itself almost overnight—just as I was trying to show Mae and Janelle a good time.

8
Due to the Coronavirus ...
Saturday, March 14

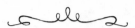

I logged onto the Guides Association of New York website about 10 a.m., checking the spreadsheet that licensed New York City tour guides were using to inform each other of what was closed and open in the city. Museums, stores, restaurants, and other points of interest were all making their own rules because the government wasn't issuing any citywide guidelines. So tour guides were relying on each other to create an up-to-date list of what remained open in the city.

I was happy to see a number of popular attractions were still open, and I began revising my plans for what I could do with Mae and Janelle, who were arriving in little more than an hour.

Oh, good, lots of attractions aren't closed yet. The Statue of Liberty is open. And Madame Tussauds wax museum is still open. I have free tickets to Madame Tussauds—maybe the girls would be interested in that.

Shutting my computer, I breathed a sigh of relief, happy to know there would be plenty to do with my nieces during their New York City vacation. Grabbing my backpack, I said, "See ya soon, Brian! I'm headed to the airport to get the girls. I'll meetcha at the pier!"

Grabbing the *New York Post* from the floor in front of our

door, I headed to the subway line that would take me to Penn Station, where I could catch the New Jersey Transit train to Newark Airport. I wasn't thrilled by the prospect of the elaborate trek, but I would rather spend eighteen dollars on public transport than seventy dollars on cab fare. And besides, I could catch up on the news during my hour-long journey.

"First coronavirus-related death confirmed in New York State," blared the headline of an article detailing the death of an 82-year-old New Yorker who had suffered from underlying health issues. I also learned that New York had more than five hundred positive cases, a jump of about a hundred cases in one day, and that "117 patients are now in hospitals." I was shocked by the increase in one day. I was also shocked to read that Disney World was planning to close—proof that a pandemic alarm was escalating all over the country.

After finishing the *Post*, I switched to news updates on my phone. Mayor de Blasio had just given a news conference, and I wasn't surprised that he had made no upcoming plans to restrict the flow of daily life. "History shows us that in crisis relatively few people have a perfect, absolutely tried and true plan," de Blasio said. "I am not ready today at this hour to say, let's have a city with no bars, no restaurants, no rec centers, no libraries. I'm not there."

That attitude made sense to me. I was still hoping that the virus would not be as bad as some people were predicting.

But then I saw that all the city's Catholic churches had decided to shut down, which prompted me to check for information about Hillsong Church, where I was planning to take the girls tomorrow for Sunday worship. I found the Hillsong website on my phone and was disappointed to see an announcement that was becoming more familiar: "Due to the coronavirus, our services have been cancelled tomorrow."

Shoot! I wanted to take the girls there because they love Hillsong's music. Well then, I'll take them to my own church, Redeemer. I'm sure it's still meeting; they said nothing about closing last Sunday.

But when I logged on to the Redeemer website, I found the same announcement that I had seen on the Hillsong site.

Wow—this is a first in Redeemer's history, I'm sure. No church service?! I never thought I'd live to see these kinds of measures. Unheard of. Unprecedented.

But my worries about closures got swept away as I arrived at Newark airport and realized I was running late. My train had taken longer than normal today, so I just concentrated on getting to the United baggage claim as quickly as possible.

"Hey! Mae and Janelle!" I yelled when I recognized the two slim figures standing slightly apart from the crowd. Running to hug them, I reached seventeen-year-old Janelle first, sweeping her up in a bear hug before turning to her fifteen-year-old sister.

"Wow, girls, you look great for waking up at, like, 5:00 a.m., right?"

Janelle answered, "Yeah, we're a little tired. Mae was able to sleep on the plane, but I couldn't."

"And you made it here alone—were there any issues?"

"None at all," Mae answered.

Whew! Thank you, Jesus! I was so worried something was going to happen. They're so young to be traveling alone. I would have NEVER considered flying on a plane at their age without an adult!

"Since it's noon, do you need something to eat?" It's a question I always ask when meeting tour groups at the airport.

"No, we ate on the plane," said Mae.

Although neither girl was very chatty, they were both smiling broadly, eagerly checking out the hustle and bustle around them. I knew they were excited to be in New York.

"Whoa—that's a *huge* suitcase for five days!" I said, ogling their waist-high black bag. "I hope you saved room for shopping!"

The girls laughed as I grabbed the suitcase and began wheeling it toward the exit. "C'mon, y'all, we're getting home very creatively—a train, a cab, and a boat—and then we walk a mile."

I laughed as their eyes grew bigger and bigger. "If ya want to save some money in this expensive town, it always involves time and energy. But we'll have fun in the process, I promise!"

Hauling the suitcase to the taxi line, we hopped into a cab. "Newark Penn Station, please."

"That'll be twenty dollahs," the cab driver growled as he peeled out of the line of taxis still waiting for a fare.

Mae looked out the window as the cabbie drove through Newark. "Why don't we just take the cab all the way into Manhattan?" she asked.

"Oh, girl, it is expensive to get there by cab—seventy dollars or more when all is said and done! We keep a tight budget, and we especially don't like to spend it on cab rides. Maybe one day if we win the lottery we'll take cabs everywhere—which would be a miracle, since we don't play." I laughed at my own joke.

Turning serious, I broached the subject of our itinerary. "Oh, I do have some yucky news, not to spoil the fun. The Broadway show we were gonna see tonight closed due to the pandemic. All of Broadway shut down only two days ago. It's such a shame that happened right before your trip. I'm so sorry!"

"Awww," muttered Janelle, sadly. Then she shrugged.

Mae asked innocently, "All right, but is Central Park going to be open?"

"Yes!" I exclaimed. How nice to be around teenagers who didn't complain at every bit of difficult news! Happy to turn back to something positive, I said, "The park is beautiful now because we're in spring. It'll be packed with folks out having fun because it's one of the nicest weekends we've had this year—everyone's busting to come out to celebrate the end of winter."

Mae asked, "Will Uncle Brian be able to join us? He's always working."

"Well, Brian has work to do today—you know it's hard to get him to step away from the desk! But he promises he'll hang with us tomorrow."

Janelle spoke up. "So then, let's do Central Park for sure tomorrow, so Uncle Brian can join us!"

Oh, good. They're not too upset. They've always been super flexible. I like to think the mission trips we took together to South Africa contributed to teaching them the importance of flexibility!

At Newark Penn Station, we lugged the suitcase up to the PATH (Port Authority Trans-Hudson) station, and I swiped the three of us in with my metro card. When we boarded the train, Janelle inserted earbuds and began listening to music. I discussed the route home in more detail with Mae. "Normally we could take this all the way into Manhattan, but it's shut down on the weekends due to construction. But at the

Exchange Place station in New Jersey, we'll board a free boat to finish the journey."

Mae brightened up when I mentioned a boat ride. "The boat will be cool!"

"Whatcha listening to, Janelle?" I asked. Janelle removed one earbud and handed it to me. "Listen to this cool song on my playlist from a French group called Polo and Pan." I was surprised by the ethereal, psychedelic sounds. "It looks like it's spinning 'round ... Lion is afraid of me ..."

"Whoa—this is what you listen to? It's super cool!" I said, trying to sound hip. Secretly, I thought it would never replace the synth-pop hits of the '80s.

Leaving the PATH station, we walked north by the river walk until we arrived at the boat loading area. "Does this boat go to Brookfield Place in Battery Park City?" I asked a dock-hand.

"Yep—taking off soon, too," he said.

"C'mon, let's hurry!" I called to the girls, walking as quickly as I could while dragging the suitcase across the pier. The girls explored the small commuter ferry as we took off, looking at the view from each window of its interior.

"There's the Statue of Liberty!" Mae exclaimed, pointing southward.

"Yes! It's pretty to look at in this gorgeous weather, isn't it?" I added, "She hasn't closed due to the pandemic yet, but you've already visited her before. Remember that when you came up eight years ago?" Mae and Janelle nodded, distracted by the beautiful view of both Manhattan and New Jersey from the middle of the Hudson River.

"You know, y'all, I take tourists to the Statue of Liberty

over a hundred times per year! I was all geared up to take a bunch of student groups to see her again this year, but apparently that's not gonna happen," I mused aloud.

"Well, at any rate," I said, changing gears, "we need to focus on the here and now. And right now we can admire her from afar and be glad she's not closed so others can enjoy her."

It took only ten minutes to cross the Hudson River, and soon the boat was docking at the terminal. As we neared the end of the metal walkway, I blurted out, "Surprise, look who's here!" pointing to Brian waiting on the sidewalk. They ran to him and the three engaged in a hugfest.

Brian's such a cuddly, loving teddy bear. I'm glad he can get away from work a bit to hang with us. He adds so much when he's around. Poor dude—all he ever does is work.

As we trekked the final mile to our apartment, we passed by a Whole Foods store, where a line snaked out the door.

"Wow, I've never seen such a long line outside that grocery store!" I marveled.

"I think they're stocking up on groceries because of the virus," Brian said.

"Well, we have a lot of food at home. I don't think we will ever have to stand in a long line like that," I mumbled.

But I grew less certain as we continued home. Sidewalks that should be full of tourists were almost empty as we passed through Tribeca and the Financial District. We saw maybe ten people, and all were clearly residents out doing errands. About half of them were wearing masks over their nose and mouth. As the girls lagged behind to take pictures, I turned to Brian, who was now lugging the suitcase. "Wow. Usually a horde of tourists would be traipsing about all over the Financial

District. Now there's no one."

"Except our brave nieces!" Brian said.

"Yes, I still can't believe they're here. A lot of parents probably wouldn't let their kid travel to New York City now with things becoming so upended, but Sean and Michelle always were intrepid parents—risk-takers in the best sense. They're no joke. They don't back down for anything! That's why Michelle is so great in the military, I'm sure."

"Yes," Brian agreed. "The kind of parents that would let their kids go on a mission trip to South Africa with *you*!"

We both laughed and watched the girls enjoy the city.

Lord, thank you for getting them here safely! Please let us enjoy our time together!

But Brian had turned serious. Keeping his voice low so the girls couldn't hear him, he said, "Christina, I watched the news right before I left to meet you all—New York State now has 613 cases, New York is at 269, and another death has been announced: a man in Rockland County."

"Wow, these numbers seem to be changing by the minute. That storm is gaining strength," I said. "But Rockland County is far from here—it seems like another world. And these are still low numbers compared to the overall population of the city and the state."

"Yeah, and the Rockland County man had underlying health issues too," Brian said.

"Well, let's keep our eye on it," I said. Although I was trying to find reasons not to panic, I was getting more nervous. Brian and I walked in silence the rest of the way to the apartment, grateful that our nieces were clearly enjoying the sights of Lower Manhattan.

Stepping inside our apartment, I announced, "Home sweet home, everyone! We've set up the sofa bed for you all—notice it's a newer sofa than when you were last here—I think two years ago? You came that day before we left for our mission trip to South Africa? Here's a little spot for your luggage so we're not all tripping over it," I instructed as I put the luggage under the foot of the pullout.

"When ya have four people in a 700-square-foot apartment, you have to get strategic to maneuver everything. Same thing with taking showers: four people for one bathroom, so we'll need to make a schedule. But we can discuss that later. Why don't we freshen up, get some snacks and coffees at Starbucks, and walk up to Chinatown and Little Italy, with a quick stop at the Brooklyn Bridge?"

"Yeah! Awesome, that would be great!"

I was happy to see that the long journey had not tired them out and happy to know I could still find things they would enjoy. Then I pointed to the pile on the table where I'd amassed a stash of cloth face masks and plastic gloves.

"I think we all should consider wearing gloves and masks," I said. "We're going to be exploring the city from one end to the other, and although you'll notice that not everyone is wearing them, maybe it's better to be safe than sorry."

I certainly wanted to make sure Janelle and Mae were as safe as possible. Even if their parents were risk-takers, I felt very responsible for their well-being while they were with me.

"Yeah, I noticed some people were wearing them in the plane, but not everyone. I'm fine to do that," Mae responded while Janelle nodded.

"I'm glad to hear that. Honestly, I should have brought

them with me so you could wear them on our way back here, but I didn't want to spring it on you in the airport.

"So let's agree to use them from now on. Just grab your masks and gloves when you're ready and we can head out!"

9

NOTHING MORE
WE CAN DO FOR YOU

Monday, March 23, Morning

I woke from a sound sleep when someone opened the door to my room. It took me a minute to figure out where I was, but I remembered quickly when a nurse appeared next to my bed. Like all the others, she was covered head to toe in protective gear.

"I brought your breakfast, along with your morning pills," she announced. "Your breakfast is pancakes and eggs. Maybe before you eat you can go ahead and take the Tylenol and hydroxychloroquine pills."

"Thank you," I said groggily.

"We have some tests to do this morning," the nurse said, as she set my breakfast on the nightstand. "Do you remember the 'sit down and stand up' test you did yesterday that measures your blood pressure?"

Yawning, I nodded and swung my feet over the side of the bed. I stood up and sat down again fast.

"Okay, now stay standing." The nurse was watching the monitor. "Wow, much better today!" she stated.

I smiled with pleasure. I was delighted to find that this effort was much easier today.

"You did so well, you can go home now, I believe!" she

chirped nonchalantly, dumping the four pills from the cups into my hand.

"Ummm, what?" I asked slowly. "Why can I go home now? I'm sick!" My voice got louder as my anxiety grew. "I'm COVID-positive! I have a sore throat; my temperature stays around 101. Just yesterday I couldn't even stand without feeling faint!" I stayed on the side of the bed, both incredulous and confused.

"Listen," the nurse said gently, as she handed me water. She waited for me to swallow the pills before she continued. "You are stabilized now. There's nothing more we can do for you at this point."

"Yes, there is," I shot back, growing bolder. "You can keep a check on my vital signs and monitor me. You can give me pain medication if I need it, and medication to make sure I don't vomit. You can give me another IV if I need it. There's plenty to keep me here!"

She waited a moment, clearly contemplating what she wanted to say. "The emergency room is the only place people suffering from COVID-19 can get care. The ER is for short-term, immediate care. That's why you can't stay here for the unforeseeable future—overcrowding is an issue, and we need the rooms for those who have life-threatening situations."

I lay back on the bed as she spoke, open-mouthed like a fish—trying to wrap my head around everything she had just told me. Why would a hospital mix COVID patients in with emergency room patients? I was no health expert, but that sure seemed strange to me!

"Someone will come check on you again soon to discuss your exit. Remember: rest, hydrate, and take Tylenol," she said, before starting her own exit routine of discarding gear and sanitizing her hands.

I thought I was in here for the long haul! I feel like I'm being kicked out—kicked out of a hospital! What in the world?!

As the nurse made her way to the hallway, I grabbed my phone and dialed Brian. "They're making me leave!"

I hit him with a long stream-of-consciousness rant.

"I know they need the bed for a future patient worse off than me—even though, according to them, this place is *not* overrun at the moment—but I also know I'm getting better care here than I could manage on my own. She says there's 'nothing more they can do for me,' but I need to be monitored! I'll bet I slide downhill right away once I leave here. I'm not healed, I'm not getting better—my blood pressure is stabilized, that's all. They're just giving me a Band-Aid and sending me off ..."

I lapsed into silence, too exhausted to continue.

Brian tried to console me, but then admitted, "I'm surprised, too. But I don't think you can fight the hospital, though. Just give me a heads-up and I'll come get you."

As I chucked the phone on the bed and began to pick sadly at my pancakes, I felt a surge of diarrhea. I maneuvered myself over to the toilet as quickly as I could, grateful that I had perfected the transfer system the day before.

Man, I'll get dehydrated again if this continues! See? Going downhill has already started.

I had just managed to get back to my bed when the door opened, and a new-to-me nurse entered, carrying a bag. "Hi, Christina! Here's some medication for you to continue the fight at home."

"Is hydroxychloroquine included?" I asked, eyeing the bag.

"Yes, it is," she said, setting it on the nightstand. "I'm going to unhook you from the blood pressure machine and take the IV needle out of your arm."

"Does it matter that I just had diarrhea? I had not had that symptom before. Would that keep me in the hospital?" I asked, as she removed my IV needle. I really did not want to leave.

The nurse paused and stared for a moment at the wall. "Hmmm. Maybe. That's worrisome. I'll talk to my supervisor about that," she said, and walked over to the trash can to begin her exit routine.

I was glad that she seemed concerned and looked forward to talking to the doctor about my new symptom. But no one ever returned to my room or called to discuss it with me.

About an hour later, the hospital phone rang. When I answered, a voice asked, "Is someone coming to get you? Just let us know when they're here, and we'll bring in someone to walk you out. That nurse will have some loperamide for you, which will address your diarrhea."

I was annoyed and frustrated but didn't feel like fighting anymore. I texted Brian and asked him to come pick me up. Still dressed in the leggings and t-shirt I had been wearing when I arrived at the hospital, I packed up everything I had taken out of my backpack in the past twenty-four hours.

Glancing at the clock, I saw it was 10:10 a.m., and I knew I had at least a half hour to kill before Brian arrived.

I decided to check Facebook to see if anyone had responded to my messages from last night. I sat back on the bed, dragged my computer out of my backpack, and balanced it on my belly. I was astonished when I opened my Facebook page.

Wow! Over six hundred likes, six hundred comments, and seventy shares! I've never seen that kind of response to any post I've ever written before.

I pored over the messages, overwhelmed by the awesome expressions of love and concern: "Oh no! I'm so sorry! Prayers for you and Brian!" "Praying, Christina! Be strong and focus on the Lord, our Great Shepherd, to carry you through!" "Oh no!! Praying for you and Brian to make complete recoveries from this terrible virus. I will put you both on our church prayer list. We love you!"

I can tell from the responses that most of my friends don't know anyone else who has COVID. Well, good—I can hog all their prayers, then! Thank you, Lord, for friends who care about us! Thank you for making me feel better. I know you know the future. Take care of all of us! Calm my nerves about being sent home!

My phone chimed, alerting me to a text message. Expecting it to be from Brian, I was surprised to find a message from Sarah, my sweet BFF of the past twenty-five years. "Christina, we want to bring food and supplies to you and Brian's family. What do you need?"

Tears sprang to my eyes as I considered how a strange twist of fate meant Sarah and Jeff were again nearby when Brian and I were in crisis. They had helped us survive the days after 9/11, giving us shelter and support in Manhattan. Now they were only a forty-five-minute drive away from where we were staying in Central Florida, ready again to offer us supplies and support.

"Thanks so much—get anything," I texted in reply. "So appreciate it. Will pay you back."

I tried to think of any specific requests I could pass on to

Sarah. I knew Sean's family would eat anything, but I had not been able to eat a full meal in almost a week. I looked up from the phone and stared ahead. "What's a good thing to eat when you don't want to eat?" I said aloud. Suddenly, I remembered how my dad had relied on Ensure, the nutrition drink, toward the end of his life. I sent another text to my sweet friend: "Ensure, Sarah—get a bunch of Ensure."

Not long after my text exchange with Sarah, Brian texted: "I'm here."

Picking up the hospital phone, I called the nurses' desk. "Okay, my ride's here and I'm ready to go. Can you send someone?"

A nurse walked into the room about five minutes later. "Follow me!"

I draped my backpack over one shoulder and picked up the bag of pills. The nurse held the doors as I walked through the anteroom and into the hallway. "This way," she said, taking the lead, as I looked around for the wheelchair I expected to be waiting for me. There was no wheelchair, and the nurse was already headed down the hall. I did not feel strong enough to walk very far, but I was going to lose sight of the nurse if I didn't get moving, so I resolved to let it go and do the best I could.

Walking very slowly, we went through the same maze of hallways I had been wheeled through the day before. As we arrived at a big set of double doors, the nurse handed me a piece of paper. "This is good information in case you need further help."

I stopped and read the paper, growing even more confused by its message. "Do you think you may have coronavirus? If so, call your healthcare provider or a virtual care provider."

The sheet listed a number of urgent-care locations in Tampa and Brandon but did not provide any information about returning to Hillsborough Hospital, which annoyed me.

If you all don't want to treat COVID patients here, then don't admit them!

I returned my attention to the paper and read to the bottom of the page: "For the safety of you and our community, please do not visit an emergency department unless you're experiencing critical symptoms or have been instructed to do so."

I looked up and told the nurse, "This is good to know, but if I get sick again I'm coming right back to Hillsborough Hospital. And since you're treating COVID patients in the emergency room, I'll be coming back here!"

She stammered, "Okay," but offered no other information or help as I walked out the double doors, still unstable and shaky and not feeling significantly better than when I had entered through the doors the day before.

10

GROCERIES AND MESSAGES AND PRAYERS

Monday, March 23, Afternoon

B rian was standing outside the car in the driveway, waiting, as I made the slow walk to him.

He gave me a hug as I got situated in the car. I asked ear-
nestly, "How are the girls and Sean? Anyone else sick yet?"

"I have been staying away from everyone as much as I can
in case they don't have it and I do, but I heard the girls have
been super tired and have exhibited various symptoms, like
short-lived sore throats and headaches. Apart from that, they
seem fine. Sean is fine so far. But I've exhibited some strange
symptoms—stomach gurgling, cramps in my arms, legs, and
stomach. Chest tightness combined with shortness of breath.
Almost like a whole inflammation in the chest area. I did a
Teladoc appointment this morning: the doctor prescribed
antibiotics and something for coughing, but I haven't really
had a cough yet. He said not to be surprised if this lasts for a
while—maybe two weeks. His patients average two weeks
with symptoms."

"Two weeks. Well, one week down, one more week to go
for me, then. I haven't had a cough yet either, praise the Lord!"
I replied. "However, let's get real, Brian—you have this, too."

I sighed. "It sounds like the girls have it as well. How could they not? We've been with them every day for the past ten days—many of those days in our 700-square-foot Manhattan apartment. I don't see how they could have dodged it!

"What if I had it before they even came, and I gave it to them? If that's true and they develop a bad case of this, I won't be able to live with myself!"

"Don't worry about that at this point," Brian consoled me. "They're okay, and I'm not sure we'll ever know how we picked it up."

"Did you ask the Teladoc for a test?" I ventured.

"Yes." Brian frowned. "He told me to just stay at home, take care of myself, and not to bother with it."

Grrrrrr ... who is getting these alleged tests? Where are they?!

My cell dinged again. A new message from Sarah: "We'll be over soon!"

Turning to Brian, I said, "Sarah and Jeff got us all some food—isn't that sweet? Looks like we'll intercept her and the groceries as soon as we get there."

"Okay," Brian said. But he sounded concerned. "Just remember we need to make sure we keep a good distance between us."

Brian pulled the car into the driveway, and as we reached the front door, a red SUV pulled up and parked at the curb, about twenty feet away. "Hi, Christina and Brian!" Sarah yelled, jumping out of the car and circling around to the passenger side. Sarah, her hair piled on top of her head and in red shirt and shorts, was a sight for my sore eyes. It had been almost six months since I had seen her, and I had to work really hard not to run to her for a big hug.

Waving, I yelled back across the front lawn, "Hey, girl!" But when she turned around, I was surprised to see a big mask covering most of her face. As Sarah unloaded bag after bag from her car and set them near the curb, I mumbled to Brian, "Geez, does she need to wear one right now? We're, like, far. It makes me feel like a freak, a leper." Then I thought about how I had almost run to meet Sarah.

Wow—what if I had run over and given her a hug? I could harm—or even kill—my best friend. What a crazy thought.

Sarah wasn't giving me that chance, though. She waved, then jumped in her car and took off.

"I'm going to text Sean that we're outside so he and the girls can isolate themselves before we come in," Brian said. "I'll bring the bags inside. You go ahead and head upstairs."

I waited until I knew that Sean and the girls were safely tucked away before entering the house. I slowly moved through the kitchen, up the staircase, and then to the bedroom to drop off my backpack. Then I headed straight to the shower.

This might be one of the longest stretches I've been without a shower in my life! This is the one situation where I'm glad I've lost my sense of smell!

I finished quickly, worried I would faint if I lingered too long in the shower.

I wrapped myself in a couple of bath towels, then made my way out of the bathroom into the bedroom and sank down on the sofa. Being clean had energized me, and I decided to start a CaringBridge account so that I could update my friends and family about my battle with the virus. I had seen friends use the online forum and knew it was a good way to share health updates without overloading everyone on Facebook.

Hmm ... I'm not sure how to start my journal entry. But I can't help thinking that as much as I love New York, this isn't the first time our lives there have been threatened. Maybe I should write about how being COVID-positive is similar to being in the city on 9/11. It's the second time NYC has exposed us to a life-threatening situation!

I chose the title for my post—"Surviving NYC, Part Deux"—and began writing.

"Hello All! Thanks for coming to the site. I'm beginning my journal referencing 9/11, because it's been hard for me NOT to tie our COVID-positive status with September 11, 2001. If you don't know our story, Brian and I were (and still are) living in the Financial District during the attacks, just six blocks away from the Twin Towers ..."

I'm really wanting to write, communicate, and connect with people right now. I need people, I need them praying for me.

I was so focused on my writing that I jumped when my phone buzzed with the peculiar chime alerting me to a Face-Time call. The smiling face of Tricia Dietz, a former mission trip teammate, filled the screen as I connected. She was calling from the Christ Church Christian Care Center orphanage in Johannesburg. "Hey, Christina!" she trilled enthusiastically. "I'm here at the 5Cs! The teenagers want to say hi to you!"

"You're still in South Africa!" I yelled with both surprise and elation. "I'm just so glad—and jealous—you were able to run over there to spend time with the children. I'd *love* to talk with them!"

Still wrapped in towels, I tried to make sure that I stayed covered and kept the screen focused on my face during this FaceTime call.

Tricia passed the phone around as twenty-odd teenagers tried to take turns peering into the screen and shouting encouragement. "I love you, Ugogo! Feel better! Hello, Miss Christina! We love you, we miss you!"

As Tricia reclaimed her phone, I said, "Tricia, thank you so much for thinking of me and assembling everyone. You made my day! I love them so much."

"Yes, Mike Sunker told the children you were feeling sick, and we've all been praying for you here. One last thing—," she said, "they want to sing for you." She panned her phone's camera over the group, now standing together in a corner of a room I recognized—the TV room of the teenage girl quarters. "Asimbonanga," they began, singing the beautiful, haunting music of Johnny Clegg, one of my favorite South African singers.

"My favorite song! They remembered!" I exclaimed.

"We love you!" the kids said together, using their hands to make heart symbols on their chests as the song ended. "We'll call you again tomorrow!" Tricia promised.

The delightfully unexpected call lifted my spirits, especially hearing the term of endearment children call me in South Africa. "Ugogo" means "Grandma" in Zulu.

After the call, I noticed a text from my old friend Tony Hale, who lives in Los Angeles. "Hey Friend! I heard you were sick! So sorry! Is there anything I can do for you?"

I replied right away. "Hey, Man! That's so sweet of you to ask! You know, I can't think of a thing right now that I need. But I'm worried about my nieces. They probably have the virus and they must be so scared. I can't even help them process it, because I'm so sick that I need to stay apart from everyone. I wish there was something *I* could do for *them*!"

Tony texted back, "I have an idea. What are their favorite shows?"

"I have heard them talk about some show called *Stranger Things* and another called *A Series of Unfortunate Events*—they love those. Why?"

"You'll see!"

Tony is a two-time Emmy winner and bona fide Hollywood superstar who starred in *Arrested Development* and *Veep*. I'm so proud of what he's accomplished—but I will always think of him first as Tone Loc, the skinny, funny kid I went to school and church with in Tallahassee.

I reopened my computer, finding more encouragement from friends who had responded to my Facebook posts. "Praying for you, Christina! God has never once left your side!" "We are praying for you here in Madagascar!" "Keep fighting. Know that there are so many prayers for you. You can beat this!!!" "20 folks here from Living Waters in LeRoy, NY praying for you today!" "I'm going to fast for you and your family's healing today."

There were comments from friends across the United States and in countries I had visited on mission trips, including India, Madagascar, and Honduras. Almost every comment mentioned prayer.

Woohoo! It's happening—people are praying for me! I'm covered in prayer!

I finally logged off the computer around 5 p.m., having spent the afternoon writing updates and reading responses on CaringBridge and my social media accounts. As I tried to stand, I was overwhelmed by a rush of body aches and rising heat, stomach indigestion, and stinging eyes. I felt I was on the verge of throwing up. I reached for the thermometer on the TV tray and took my temperature: 101. The onslaught filled me with dread. I realized it was time for another dose of Tylenol, and I hoped it could beat back these symptoms quickly.

"Brian, I'm waving! I need help!"

11

IT'S TRYING TO KILL ME

Monday, March 23, Evening

Grabbing the Hillsborough Hospital water jug from the TV tray, I began slurping steadily from the straw as I reached for the closest bottle of Gatorade with the other hand. Holding one in each hand, I began switching between the two, never setting either down, trying desperately to hydrate myself. Tears began streaming down my face, and my blood felt like it was starting to boil.

Here I go again. As soon as I start to run a temperature, I start to cry. Has to be some cause-and-effect situation.

Dashing into the room, Brian headed straight for the night-stand and announced, "Okay, I'm bringing you Tylenols." He picked up a bottle and quickly poured pills into his hand, scooted over to the fan and pointed it toward me, then set the pills on the TV tray in front of me.

"It looks like it's spinning 'round ... Lion is afraid of me." The lyrics to the song Janelle had shared with me began replaying on a loop in my mind.

Oh wow—why am I thinking about this song now? I feel completely spaced out—I think the temperature is making me high.

Brian wrapped a wet washcloth around my neck. "There, that should help. I put some ice cubes in the washcloth too," he said, turning the fan up a notch. As the cool breeze hit me, I felt bubbles moving back and forth, passing from left to right in my stomach. I pictured virus-fighting white blood cells chasing the COVID disease cells through my body, envisioning a sort of Pac-Man chase through my gurgling stomach.

Go get 'em, white blood cells!

Suddenly, fruit-punch-flavored Gatorade spewed out of my mouth with such force I was knocked prone on the sofa. I sat up and stared at a red horizontal line that streaked across the white wall of the bedroom. Horrified, I watched as the red line began to drip multiple thin vertical lines underneath it, branching out like roots of a crimson tree. Studying the mess, I followed the longest line of Gatorade, which dripped all the way behind the sofa.

Geez, how the heck did I throw up BEHIND me? Did my head just spin like Linda Blair's in The Exorcist?

Brian rushed to my side in dismay, grabbing a towel along the way. He began wiping my face and neck, but I knew I couldn't stay on the couch, as whatever was inside me was coming out both ends. Pushing Brian's hand away, I stumbled to the bucket and plopped down just as multiple waves of diarrhea rippled through my body. "It feels like my insides are coming out!"

"What do you need? How can I help?" Brian asked, kneeling on the floor beside me as I sat naked on the bucket, too weak to even try to hold the towel around me.

"Tub. Cold. Water. Bath."

I had not taken a cold-water bath since I was a kid. I hated it then and I didn't expect to enjoy it much now, but I had read that a cold bath was the quickest way to bring down a high fever. I knew my temperature had probably risen past 101; it felt like an internal fire was raging across my body.

Taking me by the arm, Brian helped me off the bucket and walked with me slowly to the tub in the bathroom right outside the bedroom. I was so sick that I didn't even bother to cover up before opening the bedroom door.

I'm walking around the house buck naked! I hope my brother-in-law and the girls aren't around. I'm sure they don't want to see me this way. They would not be able to unsee such a sight!

Carefully and slowly, I lowered myself into the tub as Brian turned on the faucet. Darts of cold water bounced off my hot skin. I began to feel nauseous again and was glad that I was already in the tub! "Brian—drinks." I pointed toward the door.

"I'll get your Gatorade and water." Brian sprinted out the bathroom door and returned in seconds. He put both drinks in my hands, and then turned off the faucet. I began taking long, deep gulps while I moved my body side to side to swish the water over my torso. I set the drinks on the side of the tub briefly to splash cold water on my arms. Brian picked up the drinks and moved toward the sink.

"No! Bring them back!" My outburst surprised both of us. I didn't have the strength to tell Brian that I could not get enough to drink. I felt like I might die if I didn't have something to swallow every few seconds. Liquids going down my throat were one of the few things that gave me comfort. But as soon as I swallowed a gulp, my throat would feel parched again, as if I had been traveling through a desert for hours with no fluids. I had never felt that sensation, and it scared me.

Don't people die of dehydration?

Brian quickly handed the drinks back to me and I relaxed a little.

The initial shock of the bathwater hitting my body had dissipated, and I was now enjoying the cold water. I sank as deep as I could into the few inches of water in the tub.

"I'm going to get you more hydroxychloroquine," Brian said, heading again for the bedroom.

"Yes, yes!" I was happy Brian had thought of the medicine. *I'll take anything and everything. I'd take cyanide if I heard it would make me better!*

Brian returned and put the pills in my mouth, and I washed them down with a sip of Gatorade and a sip of water. "Going to stand up now," I announced, holding out my drinks to Brian. I stood shakily while Brian wrapped a towel around my body. He then helped me step out and shuffle back into the bedroom, where I collapsed onto the sofa amid red-stained towels that Brian had used to wipe my vomit off the floor and the wall.

Brian's phone rang. "Hey, Sean. Yes, looks like Christina's having a bad time. Sorry if we're making so much noise."

"What?" I quizzed Brian when he set the phone down.

"Sean said he's hearing us move around a lot, and it looks like he heard you vomit. He wanted to know what's wrong— he and the girls can tell something is up."

I was mortified. I didn't want Sean or the girls to worry about me, and I sure didn't want them to see the hell taking place upstairs! Even worse, I worried that they would soon be living through a nightmare like mine.

Suddenly, my heart started beating extremely fast, thumping and bumping as if it were trying to escape my chest. I had experienced this kind of palpitation only two or three times in my life, usually after extreme exercise or fear.

Why is this happening? Am I having a heart attack? I just took the hydroxychloroquine—is it related?

After ten minutes of intermittent bursts of palpitations, my heart returned to its normal rhythm. But the scary episode had caused even more anxiety.

Brian had brought my Gatorade and water from the bathroom, and I resumed alternating gulps from each, draining the containers as quickly as Brian could fill or replace them. Every fifteen minutes I'd rush to the bucket to pee or poop. My diarrhea was unrelenting, and I felt a constant urge to throw up.

"I'm going to take your temperature," Brian said, as he put the thermometer in my mouth. A minute later he pulled it out and announced, "It's 103."

"Bath. Another bath," I whispered, although I didn't really want to expend the energy.

Brian helped me off the sofa and back to the bathroom for a cold bath, round two. Then it was back to the bedroom, where I continued the seemingly endless cycle of drinking bottle after bottle of Gatorade and jug after jug of water, then running to the bucket to lose it all.

When I retrieved my water jug from the floor yet again after returning to the sofa from the bucket, Brian blurted out, "Christina, *quit drinking!*"

"I can't do that—I'll die!" I was not being overdramatic. I believed it.

As I lifted the bottle to my lips, vomit suddenly erupted out of my mouth onto my naked body and then across the sofa. But I felt no relief from my unrelenting nausea. I began grabbing clumps of my hair, pulling it hard, seeking any sense of distraction from the pain and pressure in my stomach. Brian watched me as he sat on the bed—paralyzed and horrified.

"Brian, I have to go back to the hospital! I can't take any more of this torture!"

He shook his head. "Christina, we just left there this morning. We might drive all the way over there for them to turn you away. Let's try another bath."

After a third cold bath, an exhausted Brian walked me back to the sofa, which he had valiantly attempted to clean while I was in the bathroom.

He collapsed on the bed and pleaded, "It's been four hours of torture. Lord, please help us!" He buried his head in his hands and began to sob. I watched him, too weak to say anything aloud, but my spirit was groaning.

This can't go on any longer. Lord, help me! Holy Spirit!

This is truly a crisis. THINK. What can I do to feel better? What can I do to make this stop? Who can help me?

We had been treated by the same primary physician in New York for years, but he was thousands of miles away and it was after 9 p.m. Would he even answer the phone if we called? If I called the Teladoc service, would they tell me anything other than rest, hydrate, and take Tylenol? That was the only advice the medical professionals had offered me when I left the hospital a few hours earlier. If the hospital won't take care of me, who can I rely on?

I became convinced that I needed advice from professional people who are friends, and my brain began flipping through a mental Rolodex of all the healthcare workers we knew. Linda, Brian's cousin, a nurse. Tom, who went on one of my medical mission trips to Madagascar, a doctor. Monika, who went on a mission trip with me to South Africa, a nurse. Carlos, my long-ago college boyfriend, a pharmacist.

Carlos. Doesn't he live near here? I think he's some bigwig pharmacist at a hospital.

"Brian ... going to contact people ... maybe can help."

I labored to explain what I was doing, then picked up my computer and began typing furiously. Struggling to protect my computer from the vomit, Gatorade, water, and sweat that was dripping from my body, I used Facebook messages to send a cry for help to the friends I had identified.

Please let at least one person from this group be up and online and willing to help me out of this mess.

"Hey All, I have the virus and I'm really sick. I'm in Tampa and got back from the hospital earlier today. Should I go back to the hospital? I'm in so much pain right now. I think the virus is trying to kill me. Do you have any advice or suggestions?"

I was so relieved to see answers pouring in fast and furious from Tom, Linda, and Monika.

"Get anything with ibuprofen or naproxen—don't listen to the negative talk about it—the World Health Organization pulled back on the statement that it was harmful days ago. Take some now. 3 tablets every 6 hours."

"Only go to the hospital if you're short of breath."

"Your fecal matter is dead virus cells your body is discarding—that's great! It's leaving your body!"

"What are you taking now? Drink, DRINK."

"Relax, breathe deep."

"When you get the chance, get a pulse oximeter. That's a device that'll help you measure the oxygen level of your blood."

Someone cares. Thank you, Lord, for sisters and brothers to walk with me during this dark time!

Their words of wisdom calmed and comforted me, and I was especially enlightened by Monika's special insight:

"I know it sounds crazy, but other than IV fluids and a course of steroids for those who need ventilation, there's just no other treatment methods right now. But also, they are just so worried about spreading corona throughout the hospital to non-corona patients."

Brian followed the various instructions regarding items we had on hand, including bringing me ibuprofen and Theraflu.

I also got a message back from Carlos, even though we had not interacted personally in decades. "I don't think you should go to the hospital, but I want to hear more about your symptoms before I offer advice. Can you or Brian call me?"

I showed the message to Brian, who picked up his phone without hesitation. "Hi, Carlos, I'm Christina's husband, Brian. Nice to meet you. Please let me know if you could help us. Let me tell you what Christina's been doing the last several hours …"

Oh, my goodness. My HUSBAND is talking to my EX while I lie here sweating in a pool of fruit punch Gatorade!

I could tell Brian was getting helpful information from Carlos, and I marveled at how my past and present were colliding. I had dated Carlos for two years in the late '80s, and I had been married to Brian for the past twenty years. Carlos and I had lost touch years ago, and I only knew what he did and where he lived because we were Facebook friends. But here he was talking to my husband on a late-night call, trying to help Brian help me.

After hours of feeling under siege, I relaxed. Brian and I weren't alone anymore. We had knowledgeable people who loved us and were reaching out across the miles to offer us advice and help and support. Their support made us both feel better, and following their advice helped me get my symptoms under control.

I grew more confident that I would survive the night, and I no longer felt so alone. Thank God technology had allowed us to find a support network even when we were holed up in a guest bedroom hundreds of miles away from our doctors and the friends we would normally count on in a crisis. We certainly had never considered how isolated we could become when we made the decision to leave New York with the girls. We thought we were escaping the storm, not headed straight into the eye of the hurricane.

12
Shutting Down Around Us
Monday, March 16, Morning

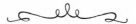

"**I**'m sorry, girls, but it looks like more of our plans are getting canceled," I explained with a frown. "We were supposed to have tea today with my friend Jenny at Alice's Tea Cup and get a behind-the-scenes tour of Fox News with my friend Lauren. However, as of yesterday, Alice's is closed, and Fox is making Lauren work from home. It's all because of the virus. I'm so sorry—I know you were looking forward to these things."

Janelle and Mae, who had not yet made it out of the pullout couch at 10 a.m., looked down but said nothing.

"Tell you what, let's go to Times Square; New York officials yesterday said that restaurants and bars have to close, but the order doesn't go into effect until tomorrow. I'll bet we can find somewhere good to eat!"

They brightened at this idea.

"And you know what? I know how you gals love Starbucks. At one point today we're gonna go to the Starbucks Roastery in Chelsea. It's the *mother* of all Starbucks!"

Janelle, normally chillaxed and too cool for school, squealed like a ten-year-old on a roller coaster, and both girls eagerly got ready to leave the apartment. Soon we were trooping across City Hall Park toward the red express train at the Park

Place station. It was surprisingly easy to make our way down underground and onto a train. "Wow, we got lucky! It's usually a lot more crowded here on a Monday morning," I told the girls brightly. But inside, I felt unnerved. It was kinda creepy to see so few people here.

The train pulled into the Times Square station fifteen minutes later, and my unease grew as I led the girls through the station to the escalator that leads to street level. Where were the crowds? Where were the street performers? As the escalator rose to 42nd Street, I saw only a few trucks traveling through the "crossroads of the world," when they were usually stacked bumper to bumper in every direction. Instead of the typical sea of tourists wandering aimlessly and gawking at the sights, about thirty people hurried by resolutely, obviously intent on taking care of their business. Everyone was wearing a mask. Trying to disguise my concern, I started pointing out landmarks.

"Look, girls! There's Madame Tussauds—the wax museum! Further down the road is a *Cake Boss* bakery—did you ever watch that reality show on TV? And that's the New Amsterdam Theatre, where *Aladdin* is playing! I know, I know—you're too old for that show." I teased. "Let's walk across the street to get into the heart of Times Square."

As we strolled up Broadway, we passed empty chairs and benches. I didn't see a single exhausted tourist guarding shopping bags. Overhead, the massive electronic billboards that give Broadway the moniker "The Great White Way" were flashing as always, unashamed that they had drawn no audience today.

"So, y'all, let's go to a popular restaurant for our brunch.

Junior's is cool—they claim to serve the best New York-style cheesecake!" I continued to act as if nothing was amiss as we turned left on 45th Street. But when we arrived at Junior's, we found a "Closed for Covid" sign taped to the front door. "Dang it!" The girls said nothing, but I could tell their frustration levels were rising. Mine was too.

Hold it together, Chris! Happy, happy—keep up the facade! The girls don't need to see your worry!

I faked a smile. "There are over 25,000 restaurants in New York City—I'm sure something is open or doing take-out!" Turning around, I saw a big sign for Buca di Beppo. Although it was not my favorite place (too touristy!), I guessed—correctly—that it would be open. As we backtracked on 45th street, we passed the Disney Store, where an employee was broadcasting to passersby, "Last day! The Disney Store closes up due to the pandemic tomorrow! Come in and see our discounts!"

Wow. It's wild to see this popular chain closing.

But as I looked around, I realized it was one of the few stores open today. Twenty percent off *Little Mermaid* merchandise wasn't enough to entice my teenage nieces, so we moved on.

I wasn't surprised by what I saw next. "Oh look—look who's here—the Naked Cowboy!" A tall, blond, tan man wearing only a cowboy hat, a guitar, and a pair of tighty-whities began to walk toward us.

"Hey," I said, turning to my nieces, "did you know I was in New York when he first came out to play his guitar in the late '90s? I remember the first time I saw him—I was twenty-eight, and here was a guy walking around in his underwear. I was sure he was gonna get arrested!"

They laughed as we stood for a few minutes, watching him badly strum a few chords and strike poses for a phantom audience. I couldn't figure out why he would even be here today—there was no one in Times Square to tip him or take pictures with him—his *raison d'etre*. The three of us and a few lonely buskers and costumed characters had the streets to ourselves.

"An empty Times Square. On a beautiful spring day. It would normally be packed," I said, thinking out loud. "I bet you will never see it like this again," I told the girls, trying to stay positive—at least outwardly. Inwardly, I knew I had seen Times Square look this empty on only one other occasion.

This looks just like it did after 9/11. I never thought I'd see New York City look this empty again. It's really ominous. The world seems completely backwards right now.

After lunch at Buca, where we were almost alone in the cavernous restaurant, I had an idea. "I have free tickets to Madame Tussauds wax museum—the place we passed earlier. Do you want to go there?"

Both immediately frowned at the suggestion but were too polite to verbalize their answer. Reading their reactions loud and clear, I had another option up my sleeve.

"There is something we haven't done in the city that is cool and is open—it just requires walking. Have you ever heard of the High Line?"

"No," Janelle answered. "What's that?"

"It's an old elevated railroad that has been converted to a park. It's a thirty-foot-tall, one-and-a-half-mile trail, and it's got the neatest landscaping and artwork on it. It also has a super-cool view of the city and goes through hip neighborhoods like Chelsea and Greenwich Village."

"That sounds fun!" Mae confirmed.

"Okay," I said. "We'll take the subway to a stop called Hudson Yards—a new area in town that's also cool to see. Remember to get your masks and gloves," I said, grabbing mine off the restaurant table and leading us toward the purple 7 subway line. There weren't many other riders, and all were wearing masks and gloves, like we were. No one spoke, and I noticed people stealing furtive glances at each other.

"People seem paranoid," Janelle whispered, as we exited. I tried to find some reassuring words, but I knew they wouldn't be genuine.

We arrived at street level after a very long, steep escalator ride, and I looked around. What was usually a chaotic mix of construction workers, tourists, residents, and office workers was so bare today that it felt apocalyptic. Trying to remain upbeat, I said excitedly, "This way!" pointing toward a patch of tall, ultra-modern glass buildings and a seven-story, million-square-foot mall. As we approached the courtyard in the midst of these buildings, Mae stopped dramatically. "What is that?" She pointed toward a massive structure that resembled a wicker wastebasket.

"Oh, that's the Vessel! It's a combination of an observatory, an obstacle course, and an architecturally super-cool attraction that's the new big thing in town. You can go up in it and walk around. People say they love the view of the Hudson from it."

"Have *you* gone up in it yet?" Janelle asked.

"I'm embarrassed to say I haven't—I've been too busy to reserve the special online tickets, and it's always packed." I looked around the deserted courtyard. "Well, it's *normally* totally packed. I'm sure it's closed, just like everything else is."

As we skirted the Vessel en route to the High Line, a man appeared and called to us with a very un-New York–like exuberance. "You want to come up?" I looked around to see if he was talking to someone else, but we were the only ones in the courtyard.

I approached the mask-wearing gentleman. "It's open?" I asked. "We can just go right up with no ticket?"

"Sure, no one's here!" he said enthusiastically. "C'mon in!"

I looked at the girls, who were nodding eagerly. "All right, let's do it! I'm experiencing something for the first time in New York City—I'm a tourist in a town where I guide tourists! Ha—this is great!"

We stepped into a small glass elevator that slowly carried us to the Vessel's sixteenth floor. We exited the elevator and were immediately surrounded by a breathtaking cityscape view. All three of us squealed in delight.

"Wow—look at that! Gorgeous! You couldn't get more of a 'New Yorky' view," I gasped, spinning to take in all of the 360-degree view. To the south, old red-brick warehouses from the Meatpacking District peeked through tall glass buildings. The Hudson River flowed to the west of us, and behind the Hudson was a brilliant blue sky set against the backdrop of New Jersey's rocky coast. To the north, I could see the Jacob K. Javits Convention Center and the southern end of Hell's Kitchen. The massively tall modern towers of the brand-new Hudson Yards district filled in any gaps.

"You know, ladies, many of these buildings are residential. Wouldn't this be an interesting area to live in? There are people living all up on those floors," I said, pointing at the tall buildings of Hudson Yards that surrounded us.

"Yes, sure! Totally!"

Suddenly, we heard a lot of shouting and began looking for the source. "What's going on? Who's yelling?" I asked. "It's a dude, clearly—one man. He's in one of these nearby buildings, on a balcony or maybe yelling out of a window. I can't see where the sound is coming from. I can't really understand him either. What do you think he's saying?"

"I think he's yelling, 'Go home,'" Janelle said.

The shouts grew louder and louder, and it became clear the man was directing his rants at the three of us. We scanned the nearby buildings but could not pinpoint the source of the voice. But we no longer had any doubt what he was saying: *"Go home! Go home!"*

His tone was urgent, angry, unkind, and insistent—an unseen force warning us of what we could not yet begin to fathom.

"He's yelling at us—some strange guy is telling us to go home," Mae declared.

I get it—the message is loud and clear. We shouldn't be here. The reality of the situation is impossible to ignore. Clearly, fun-time in NYC is OVER. The New York we know and love is gone for now. It's time to pull the shade down on everything that makes the city vibrant and go hibernate. Okay, okay, dude! We're GOING!

"Ladies, have we seen enough?" I asked, wanting to move us out of the line of negativity being sent our way. They nodded, and we hiked down the hundred-and-fifty-foot structure in subdued silence, then continued toward the High Line entrance from the Hudson Yards courtyard. The on-ramp to the High Line was blocked by a tall chain-link fence bearing a sign: "Due to COVID, the High Line is closed."

"Seriously? I didn't even know the High Line *could* close," I said, defeated and frustrated. "C'mon, girls, let's go back home. It's time to leave."

We turned on our heels and crossed back through the Hudson Yards courtyard. Before we stepped onto the escalator that would carry us down to the subway, Janelle asked enthusiastically, "Are we gonna go to the Starbucks?"

I had forgotten about my Starbucks promise, but Janelle certainly had not!

I looked at my watch: 3:15 p.m. "Sure, let's do that thang! We need to take a quick cab ride, though, because the subway is far from where that Starbucks is." We walked a block to 34th Street, where I hailed a cab with ease.

"15th and 9th, please!"

The cabbie shot across 34th Street and then down 9th Avenue. The drive took only took ten minutes because there was so little traffic on the road.

We stepped out of the cab and faced a huge double-height set of wooden doors. "Right in here, ladies!" Leading us into the Starbucks, I could hear Janelle and Mae gasp behind me.

"I know! It really is quite a sight, isn't it? Have you ever seen a three-story, 23,000-square-foot Starbucks?" I looked back and saw them standing stock-still, eyes big, mouths open.

"This is *awesome*," Mae raved.

"You know, there are only a few of these in the world." Ever the tour guide, I pointed out the cool decor, such as the pipes lining the ceiling, the fireplace, the store, and the five separate bars for ordering in the cavernous space. It was packed, with people waiting in long lines at each station.

"Aha! So *here's* where everyone's been hiding!" I joked,

looking around at all the hip millennials in line waiting to order their expensive lattes.

"I tell you what, ladies, find a menu and stand in line. I'm actually in the mood for my favorite drink, kombucha, and I need to use the restroom. I'm going to go across the street to Chelsea Market and accomplish both tasks, especially since I know exactly where to get my favorite brand. I'll meet ya back here," I said.

I crossed the street and entered Chelsea Market, a food and shopping emporium where I loved to bring tourists, expecting it to be as packed as Starbucks. But I was practically alone. As I headed for the staircase leading to the basement restrooms, I passed shuttered stores and empty food kiosks. After using the restroom, I returned to the main floor and breathed a sigh of relief when I found my kombucha store open. Making my way back to Starbucks, I came to a quick and definitive conclusion:

We have to leave New York right now. All of us. Now. I can't stand seeing the city like this. And although some places seem unaffected, like the Starbucks, they can't make up for the ghost towns in other areas. The pending doom is just—there. It's tangible.

I collected the girls, and we headed home. Back in the apartment, I cornered Brian in the bedroom and shut the door behind us. "Brian," I whispered, "it's time for the girls to leave New York. The city is shutting down around us. Restaurants aren't open, shops have closed—all we can do is walk around, and there's a limit to doing even those things. It's creepy outside—it looks like the apocalypse has happened! People have deserted the streets and are holed up inside. Someone even yelled at us to 'go home' while we were having fun on the Vessel! And the atmosphere is really off-putting—there's a demonic element in the air."

Brian looked skeptical.

"Okay, maybe that's being too dramatic. But I definitely feel an oppressive energy. It's scaring the girls, I think. It's worrying me, too. The fear of this virus and the city's reaction to it went from slightly concerned to terrified in a sprint, with no in-between. It snuck up on me, too. You've been working at home—you haven't seen what it looks like out there. It's a ghost town. Let's book them on the next flight back to Tampa."

"Really?" asked Brian, surprised, when I finally paused for a breath. "When we went to Central Park yesterday it was filled with people!"

"That's because it's one of the only places people can go and socially distance! You can't keep New Yorkers trapped in their small apartments forever! I know what you mean, but I think seeing all those people yesterday lulled us into a false sense of normalcy. And it wasn't just Central Park that seemed normal. Yesterday we walked over the Brooklyn Bridge, ate at the Clinton Street Bakery in DUMBO, had chai tea at the Chai House on Mott Street, shopped at Mystique in SoHo. All that was open, and there were other people in these places besides us, too. But even yesterday, remember when we tried to go to the observatory at the Top of the Rock and it was closed? And nobody was exploring Rockefeller Center and there was hardly anyone in Union Square.

"I think I've been so focused on being a good host to the girls that I've only been paying attention to what is still open instead of realizing how much is closed, how few people are around, and how the city changed on a dime."

Brian was not completely convinced. "But you're still working for the Marriott, right? Surely they would tell you if you aren't supposed to work next week."

"You're right," I admitted. "I haven't heard that the Marriott is closing or terminating my job or anything. But from what I saw today, there is no way I'm going to be leading tours. There are so many mixed messages these days. It's all been so confusing! But, Brian, I'm not confused about this anymore. We have got to get the girls back home. And I think we need to leave too."

As he raised his eyebrows, I said, "Hear me out. I know the girls made it up here alone fine, but after these strange last few days I know they'd appreciate it if we accompanied them home. And we *can*. Redeemer is letting you work remotely, and except for the Marriott, all my other work has been canceled or put on hold. We don't have any particular reason to stay here. And remember that article we read—the one about the virus and survivors of 9/11? I think it will be a while until the virus gets to Manhattan, but if it does and we get it, according to that *New York Post* article, we might experience more serious complications. We can't take any chances."

"That's true," Brian concurred. "And if we go with the girls to Florida, we could stay a week or so at my brother's and catch up with him. Maybe we could go visit your mom in Tallahassee and then spend some time at the beach in the Panhandle until things get back to normal in New York. That shouldn't be too long—maybe a few weeks?"

"Great idea!" My excitement grew as I imagined a short break from the rat race. "We'll make a vacation out of it. I'll take leave from the Marriott—people aren't coming to NYC anyway—and we'll just use this as a short breather from New York. The Lord knows we need it!"

Although I was unnerved by my day in the city, now I was excited. *We had a plan.* And an extended vacation sounded glorious.

This is so great—I get to take a break from my life, which I so need. Lord, THANK YOU for this opportunity. Burning the candle at both ends for as long as I have has done a number on me. Maybe this will refresh me. Get me back on track. Get me excited about life and all the wonderful things you've brought our way that have become a burden rather than a blessing because I'm too dang tired to enjoy it!

Brian reached for his computer. "I'll book the first flight possible tomorrow."

13
ABOUT LAST NIGHT
Tuesday, March 24, Morning

"Christina? You okay?" Brian was shaking my arm. "You haven't moved much in the past few hours. I wanted to make sure you're—," he hesitated. "Alive," he said, his voice trailing off.

Squinting at the light streaming in the windows, I looked down and discovered my legs were draped over the sofa armrest. "I guess I fell asleep on the sofa?" I sat up and caught sight of the alarm clock: 6:08 a.m.

The carnage of the night before was on full display around me. Red Gatorade had dried on the wall behind the sofa. Crumpled towels were amassed in piles all over the room, and several featured big red stains. Empty Gatorade bottles and water jugs were strewn throughout the bedroom. Patches of dried red vomit dotted my legs and torso. The bucket was perilously close to overflowing with vomit, pee, and excrement, needing to be emptied. Looking at the bucket, I knew I didn't have the energy to empty it and that Brian didn't either.

Thank goodness I can't smell it!

Brian reached over to the bookcase and opened a bottle of Ensure. "You need to get some nutrition, Christina," he said, and handed it to me. "How do you feel?"

Sipping the Ensure, I assessed myself. "Throat hurts. No

fever. Feel weak. My body is like, 'What the hell?'"

"How is your breathing?"

"Not great," I said. "Feel more congested." I coughed deliberately, wanting to know how my lungs would react. I was alarmed by a hint of rattling mucus. "Hear that?"

Please, Lord—not the lungs! I've read how the ventilator is helping COVID patients, but it seems painful. I don't want to go down that road. Protect my lungs, Lord!

"Brian," I said slowly, painfully. "Can't have another night like last night. The COVID bugs were working hard to kill me. No more."

Nodding, Brian stared at the floor. His haggard face showed the strain of last night's nightmare. He had not been feeling well himself, and he had spent most of the night caring for me.

"Thank goodness for your friends, though, and my cousin Linda," he said. "They really came through last night; that was some of the best advice we've gotten so far. We're going to become amateur COVID-19 experts by listening to them."

I wondered how many people had died with this virus because they didn't have anyone to help them or to give them advice like I got last night. Obviously, doctors and hospitals can't take care of everyone right now—I was proof of that! We were going to have to take care of each other.

Brian's phone rang, and he stepped across the room to retrieve it from where it was charging.

"Hi, Sean." He paced while listening to his brother, saying very little. He hung up and sat down heavily on the bed. "Sean said he woke up feeling bad. He's having the same issues I've experienced—shortness of breath and chest tightness. He called Teladoc."

I stared at the red-stained wall. "Wow. He really has it too. Are he and the girls going to get tested?"

"No, he said the doctor discouraged it. Said it's pointless. The doctor told him just to hunker down and take care of it at home."

"Hmmm," I said, making a face. "Yuck." The "don't test" advice annoyed me.

Why wouldn't we test everyone? I want my family to be counted in statistics, to know their status for sure, and to have accurate medical records verifying their medical history.

"How do you feel?" I asked.

"Oh, I'm okay," Brian responded wearily. "I'm feeling fine. Just worried about you. I think I'll go take a shower after I dump this bucket."

The exhaustion in his voice frightened me.

Lord, I'm draining Brian of all the fight he has in him for me, when he needs it for himself! I'm weakening him! What's going to happen when we both have nights like last night? We'd need someone to take care of both of us. Oh Lord, please help us!

Fighting my growing anxiety, I decided to check for new emails or social media posts, hoping I would find some well wishes to cheer me up. Opening my computer, I was surprised to find fifty new emails. I began clicking on each of them. "Christina, what's going on? Are you still in the hospital?" "How are you and Brian and the family?"

Wow, my friends and family all want updates—they seem really worried. Might be a good time to write a CaringBridge blog.

I clicked onto the CaringBridge site and typed in the subject line "About Last Night." The CaringBridge site helped me feel less isolated, and writing about my experience gave me something to do other than think about my symptoms. After I composed an update, I checked my texts, and found a message from my friend Maxine.

"Do you think you had the virus when you were here? Should I go get tested?"

I felt my cheeks grow hot. I hadn't seen Maxine in weeks!

Is everyone I contacted and asked for prayer calculating the last time they saw me and worrying about whether I gave the virus to them? Do I need to add details about when I got sick and the coronavirus incubation period to every email update? Am I gonna be a social pariah over this thing?

I texted back, "Maxine, I last saw you at Bible study March 2, and I didn't have the virus then. If you have symptoms, go get checked out (don't be surprised if you're not allowed a test. Despite what you're hearing in the media, they're hard to get). But if it turns out you have it, you DIDN'T get it from me."

I sat back and thought about my friend. Maxine, who was about seventy, had diabetes and had been a heavy smoker at one point in her life. I worried that she would get the virus easily if she was exposed to it and might get very ill—or worse. My emotions were bouncing wildly: I was worried about what this virus could do to Maxine and other friends; angry because I felt I had been accused of spreading it; sad that I was making people nervous; guilty that I might have made my family sick; heartsick because I was far away from my beloved New York City home and friends; scared because I didn't know what this virus was going to do to me next.

As I tried to process all my emotions, I kept pausing to scratch my back. Finally, reaching under my t-shirt, I felt bumps across my lower back. I made my way as quickly as I could to the bathroom and twisted around to try to look in the mirror.

"Brian! Look at my back!" I exclaimed.

Sensing my urgency, Brian turned off the water and stepped out of the shower, throwing a towel around him as he crossed the room to examine my back, which had erupted into one huge rash. Tiny red itchy bumps stretched from my shoulders to my hips.

"You had a bad allergic reaction to something," he said.

"To what?" I asked, staring at my back in the mirror. My eyes shifted from my back to my face, and I gasped. "Brian, look at my lips!"

My lips were swollen. They hadn't felt any different, but I could see they were plumped up.

Brian studied them and agreed. "Yes, there is a small difference. I hadn't noticed because they weren't huge and hadn't changed color."

I rushed back to the sofa, grabbed my computer, and messaged Linda, Brian's cousin, to ask her advice about my back and lips. She answered immediately, and I read her message aloud to Brian.

"It sounds like angioedema—a swelling beneath the skin. Must be an allergic reaction to something—probably medication."

"I don't know," Brian said pensively. "But it might be best for you not to take any more hydroxychloroquine pills for now. I mean, you were only taking that and Tylenol, and I don't think Tylenol can do this to your lips and back."

I felt more worried than before. The hydroxychloroquine was the only medicine that might have an effect against the virus. The FaceTime ringtone interrupted the latest drama.

"Hey, Christina! It's Tricia and the 5C girls calling from South Africa again!" Tricia's huge smile filled the screen, but I didn't share her excitement today.

"Hi, Tricia!" I said weakly, mustering a smile. Studying my face, Tricia quickly became subdued. "Tricia," I whispered in my gravelly voice, "I had a bad night last night. I can't talk long." Her smile looked as forced as mine felt.

"Well, Christina, the girls just want to say a quick hi. You seem—strong!" But she could not hide the fear in her eyes. The phone was passed around to the teenagers, who offered loud, happy well wishes.

"Thanks, girls." I tried to muster whatever strength I had. "I love you!" Their beautiful faces usually spark so much love and joy in my heart, but today, that joy was like a distant, apathetic memory. I felt as if I were looking at them from a tunnel that was carrying me farther and farther away. It was as if my heart and mind had begun a process of shutting down, disentangling me from anything and anyone I loved and felt connected to.

Tricia returned to the phone and said, "Good talking to you, Christina. We'll continue to pray for you!"

Tricia's stunned and forlorn look were the last things I saw as the phone disconnected.

"Brian, there's no more Gatorade. I drank it all. What do we do?" I said, looking at the scores of empty bottles lining the floor.

"Well, that leaves us in a tough spot, because none of us can go anywhere and get anything because it's clear we're all COVID-positive."

"What about delivery? From a grocery, CVS ... ?"

Picking up his computer, Brian spent several minutes clicking away, growing increasingly frustrated. "Looks like deliveries from anywhere will take at least a week!"

"Wow—a delivery taking a week to get here. Who could have imagined that even a couple of weeks ago?"

"Yeah, and I've read that thermometers, Tylenol, and toilet paper are almost impossible to come by—even if you can get to a store. Who would have thought it in this day and age?" Brian said as he continued to search online for a delivery service.

I didn't want to ask Sarah to drive all the way over again, but I knew we desperately needed supplies. I picked up my computer to see if I could find a friend who lived in the area.

Man, if I were in New York City or Tallahassee, I'd have a bunch of people who could help. I'm pretty far away from my circle of support, though.

I scanned the hundreds of comments on a recent Facebook post, and one from Stephanie Prince jumped out at me: "I live nearby, Christina. Call me if you need anything!" I hadn't really talked to Stephanie since college, but she might be just the lifeline I needed.

In a private message, I wrote, "Stephanie, I'm in a pickle—I need a few things from the grocery store/pharmacy, and no one from my household can get out to get it, and deliveries everywhere are backed up by several days. Can I take you up on your offer to help? Sorry to be a trouble … "

She responded almost immediately. "I'm so concerned about you! Just let me know what you need, and I'll take care of it. I'm about a half hour from you."

That's awesome. God, thank you for blessing us! You're showing your grace and mercy through the kindness of others!

Looking over Facebook and CaringBridge comments, my heart began to awaken from its increasingly deadened state. The love and concern expressed by friends and acquaintances pulled me out of the brain fog I had been descending into. I posted a comment to Facebook:

This virus is teaching me a lesson on gratitude, something I'm really not good at day to day. I'm grateful I'm better now than I was last night. I'm grateful Brian is not worse. I'm grateful for all the well wishes, including my Skype calls with the children of the 5Cs orphanage in Johannesburg the past 2 days. Grateful for Sarah, who brought me and Brian tons of food yesterday (and left it safely outside the door). Grateful for the place where we are staying and for the family we're staying with—that they are holding steady. There's a lot to be grateful for. Thank you, Jesus!

While I was typing, Brian stretched out on the bed. "I'm going to take a nap—last night was exhausting."

"Me too," I said. I finished my post and shut my laptop, then shuffled from the sofa to the bed. "How many hours did that go on?"

"About six," Brian mumbled wearily. "Longest night of my life."

"Thank you, Brian. You saved my life last night. I love you," I said, close to tears, as I snuggled up to him.

One thing is for sure—if Brian hadn't been there to take care of me, I believe that would have been my last night on earth.

Brian was always so calm and level-headed and so good at keeping me grounded. And he always knew how to make the

best of my impulsive ideas—like leaving New York City at a
moment's notice.

14

Looking for a Test

Monday, March 16, Evening

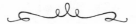

"All set," Brian said, spinning away from his computer. "I changed the girls' flights from Wednesday to tomorrow, and I got us tickets on the same flight. We will be flying out of Newark at 2:15 tomorrow afternoon."

I was glad he had been able to get tickets and also glad we would not be leaving super early the next day.

"Since you were with the girls again today," Brian said, "I'll take them out tonight to the South Street Seaport and we'll spend some quality time. I'll talk to them then about the flight change."

"Great! Way to step up, Uncle Brian!" I laughed. "I think they'll be totally fine with the change of plans; they're super flexible and we're tired from all our walking the past few days. I think they're mentally drained as well."

"You rest," Brian urged, as I opened the bedroom door to rejoin the girls, who were watching TV in the living room. "Okay, ladies, you're going out tonight with Uncle Brian—just the three of you. Why don't you all get ready?"

"Awesome!" Mae replied. Janelle said little but flashed a dazzling smile. Quality time with Brian is a prized commodity.

"Okay, Christina," Brian called, "we're off—see you soon!"

"Bye, y'all!" As the front door closed, I sank down onto the sofa and closed my eyes, but images of empty streets, fear-ful glances, shuttered stores, and empty restaurants filled my mind. And I could still hear the stranger's voice: "Go home!"

I'm so relieved we are leaving tomorrow. I'm sure this is the right move.

Suddenly energized by the thought of escaping the city, I hopped up and made a beeline to the bedroom. "I'd better pack!" I said aloud. Rooting around in my closet, I tried to imagine what I would need to take on our brief and sponta-neous mini-vacation.

We're not going to be gone long. Maybe a few weeks? We'll be in Florida—it will be hot; we will probably go to the beach. But I really don't need anything bigger than my backpack. I have some clothes I keep at Mom's that I can pick up when we get to Tallahassee.

I grabbed my backpack and shoved in a few pairs of under-wear, a pair of shorts, a few t-shirts, a pair of leggings, a swim-suit, and a pair of flip-flops. Seeing my Bible on the nightstand, I tossed that in along with my Amy Carmichael book, excited that I would finally have time to finish that monster book. As I finished packing, I realized we were getting ready to get on a plane and wondered if it was actually safe to fly right now. One infected person without a mask could endanger all of us!

Then I started wondering about myself. I didn't feel sick, but as a tour guide, I had been all over the place the last few weeks—touring and talking and riding the subway and paint-ing the town red. It would be a smart idea to get a clean bill of health before I climbed into a plane.

I decided I would walk to a Downtown hospital to get tested for COVID. The hospital was just down the street, so I thought I could get there and back before anyone knew I was gone. In fact, we lived so close to the hospital that I often joked with Brian, "If something happens to me, don't bother to call 9-1-1; just throw me onto our lobby's luggage cart and wheel me down the street!"

I threw on my black coat, grabbed my mask, and headed out, passing no one during my short walk. Although the narrow, historic streets of the Financial District are rarely busy in the evenings, it was jarring to feel like I was alone in a city of almost nine million people. I walked through the sliding glass doors of the hospital's emergency room entrance. An elderly woman sleeping in a shabby chair in the run-down lobby was the room's only occupant. I headed toward a woman behind a small reception desk. She watched me approach, her eyes wary above her mask.

"Hey—do you all offer COVID tests? I'd like to get tested for the virus," I felt like I was shouting so she could hear me through my mask.

"Oh no. We have no testing here," she responded with a dismissive tone and a wave of her hand.

Slightly annoyed, I responded, "Oh, I assumed that all hospitals in New York City have tests. Well, do you know where I can get one?"

"I don't know, not many places in town have them." She began asking me questions in a rapid-fire monotone. "Do you have any symptoms? Are you feverish? Do you have a sore throat? Do you feel like you have the flu?"

"No," I said. "None of those. But I'm about to take a plane ride. Shouldn't I get checked out, just as a precaution?"

"Just wear a mask. You don't have any symptoms, so I don't have anything else to offer you. If you have any other questions, direct them to the CDC," she instructed, pointing at something behind me.

I turned and saw a poster mounted on an easel near the sliding doors, which I had missed when I entered: "Updated Visiting Guidelines." I headed for the poster, grateful to finally get some *official* information! I read every line, looking for something related to my situation, but the entire poster was announcing new restrictions on hospital visitors. At the very bottom of the poster, there was a line that stated, "For more information on COVID-19, visit www.cdc.gov or nyp.org/coronavirus-information." I looked back at the receptionist, but she had already dismissed me and gone back to typing at her computer.

Defeated, I exited the sliding doors and trekked back up the dark and deserted street to my building. I resolved not to tell anyone about this little waste of time.

See? I'm making a big brouhaha over nothing. Just get out of here, go to Florida, relax, and enjoy yourself. You deserve a break.

I slowed as I got closer to my building and took a deep breath, secretly relieved I didn't have to get jabbed or swabbed or whatever they did to test for the virus. However, the visit to the Downtown hospital had disturbed me. I had heard the president say on the news that there were plenty of tests. If that was true, then where were the tests? I thought I was doing the responsible thing by trying to get tested before I got on a plane. If the virus was so bad, shouldn't we all have been getting tested so we knew whether we should stay away from everyone else?

But maybe the fact that I couldn't find a test was actually good news. If the major hospitals in New York City didn't have tests, could the virus really be that bad? New York City is usually at the forefront of everything, and the rest of the country follows suit. If this city didn't have tests, then who would? Maybe testing was not so important.

When I got home, Brian and the girls were still out. An early-to-bed/early-to-rise person, I was exhausted from trying to adapt to teenage sleep preferences for the past few days, so I took this chance to slip into bed before they got home. I went to sleep grateful that the three of them were enjoying their last night in the city and looking forward to time in sunny Florida.

15
GOING DOWNHILL
Wednesday, March 25, Afternoon

I opened my eyes and propped myself up in bed so I could see the clock—it was a little after noon. I had slept past the time for my next dose of Tylenol. Sure enough, my face felt flushed and my throat felt parched, sure signs that my fever was rising. I felt spaced-out and high, and I only wanted to lie on my back, disentangle myself from my surroundings, and retreat into my mind.

But I forced myself to get out of bed and move to the sofa. Waves of nausea washed over me as I threw back some Tylenol pills that were sitting on the TV tray. I began drinking water as if I were preparing for war and tried not to scratch my back.

Stirring in the bed, Brian murmured, "Do you need anything?"

"No," I said between gulps. "But starting to go downhill. Just so you know."

He groaned and turned to face me. "I'm so sorry, Christina."

Brian got out of bed. He headed toward me with the thermometer and put it in my mouth. "101," he reported.

I began focusing solely on ingesting liquids and relieving the pressure in my abdomen, shutting out everything else. Tylenol. Liquids. Sleep. Repeat. It's all I had done for the past twenty-four hours. Thankfully, I had not descended back into the depths of Monday night's horrors, but I knew I was losing ground in my fight against this virus.

My mind spun randomly. I mulled over the results of a recent Enneagram test I'd taken: I am a Seven, "The Enthusiast." Sevens are a "busy, variety-seeking type, spontaneous, versatile, disorganized." I began analyzing each attribute, pondering examples from my life that affirmed or disproved my "Seven-ness." Meanwhile, the lyrics of the song Janelle had shared with me played in my head: "It looks like it's spinning 'round ... Lion is afraid of me."

At some point, I realized Brian was speaking to me.

"Christina, you've been out of it for hours. Are you okay?" He was bending down in front of the sofa, his face inches from mine. "Is there something I can get you?"

I looked up at the clock: 3:00 p.m.

Had I been sitting here for almost three hours?

I shrugged, too tired, detached, and foggy to speak.

"Christina, you've got to *fight*," Brian begged.

I didn't have the strength to answer him, but internally, I was screaming.

What do you mean—fight? What do you think I'm doing right now? What else am I supposed to DO to fight?

I tried to rouse myself from this brain fog. Maybe reading a book would help me focus. Looking around the room, I spotted the massive book I had brought with me about Amy Carmichael, the missionary to India. Sliding it toward me, I spied its title: *A Chance to Die*. I chucked it back on the bookshelf like it was poisonous and then slumped back on the sofa.

I'm not reading THAT. Stupid virus ruined a perfectly good book!

Picking up my computer, I checked on my social media posts, emails, and CaringBridge responses. I was a bit surprised to find lots of "advice" for fighting COVID—and became annoyed by many of the suggestions.

"Christina, make sure you drink ginger ale and eat popsicles—that will make you feel better!"

"Make sure you get vitamin C, Christina!"

"Don't take Advil or ibuprofen! I read that it's bad for you!"

"You need Juice Plus products!"

Wow, everyone has a cure for COVID! Everyone's at home watching TV or getting tips from their Twitter feed or Facebook friends. But there's so much conflicting information out there—who should we listen to? What advice should we follow? I mean, even the experts don't seem to have the answers, so why do so many people without any experience in health care (who have never had the virus!) seem to think they know everything?

And anyway, where do people think I can get my hands on all this stuff? I guess everyone is so used to thinking they can pop out and buy anything they want. But none of us can leave the house right now, and deliveries are taking forever. And even if we could leave the house, most of the stores around here are completely sold out of Gatorade and ginger ale and chicken soup and vitamin C—and lots of other things! We're in a new normal, y'all!

I realized that social media had become a double-edged sword. I was so grateful to have been able to reach out to so many people so quickly, and the loving comments, good wishes and prayers truly provided me hope and strength. But it was also a place where people tossed out rumors and peddled unproven cures and argued with anyone who dared to disagree.

I'm so, so glad this type of social media did not exist during 9/11.

That would have made an almost unbearable situation even worse. Everybody would have been speculating about the terrorists' identities and sharing endless theories about how they got onto the planes and placing blame for why it had happened and posting warnings about more terrorists and their next targets. All of it would have just stirred up confusion, anger, and bad feelings toward each other and toward our government—which was exactly what was happening now.

Personally, I wished more people would look for ways to provide us with groceries or supplies, rather than just offering advice without knowing more about my symptoms or what I was doing for them. Prayers and good wishes and sympathetic messages were welcome, too, but I didn't want to be bullied through cyberspace.

Gale, a childhood friend, had left a private message that initially made me cringe:

Christina, I just read your "About Last Night" post. Please go back to the hospital. They need to be taking care of both you and Brian. That is their JOB. If they won't take you at that particular hospital, go to a different one. This is why we have healthcare providers—to help us when we are sick. Please go back to the hospital today. Do not let them turn you away.

She's got a point, I guess. But they probably WILL turn me away. And do I really want to be back in the hospital: the IV needles, the painful tests, the doctors and nurses under all those protective layers? Not to mention the energy I'd expend just getting there. And am I ready for them to really find something wrong and do something like intubate me or hook me up to a ventilator?

My phone rang. I picked it up but set it back down when I saw it was my mom calling. I knew I didn't have the energy to talk to her, and I didn't want her to know the extent of my misery. I let the call roll to voicemail, then texted, "No worries, Mom, I'm fine. Will call later."

I returned to social media and scrolled past a popular article that many of my contacts had shared: "At least 50 priests killed by coronavirus."

Wow—I'm praying for the Lord to get me through this, but I'll bet these priests prayed for the same thing. If their prayers went unanswered, is that how God will answer mine?

Another article gave the latest statistics for New York: "17,800 cases have been confirmed in New York City, with 199 deaths. The city's infection rate is five times higher than the rest of the country, and its cases are one-third of total confirmed US cases."

I had no clue the virus was so widespread when I was walking around with the girls, drinking expensive chai tea in Chinatown and shopping with them in SoHo. I feel like a bonehead.

Reading and reasoning were beginning to give me a headache, and I didn't have the energy to fully respond to anyone. I shut the computer, feeling like I was retreating and regressing into my own mind.

I coughed deliberately and was sure I could hear phlegm rattling more aggressively than it had yesterday. That one cough brought on a full-on coughing spell, and I began worrying that I could have pneumonia. My back itched constantly, and I couldn't stop myself from clawing at it. I picked up a small compact and looked in the mirror and saw that my lips were still swollen.

It's 4:30 p.m. I'm really scared—am I heading for another night like Monday night? This was about the time when my body started going to war that night. Lord, please spare me two things—another terrible episode like Monday night and a ventilator! Please, Lord!

"Christina, *fight!*" Brian was standing over me, imploring me.

How long has he been standing there? Have we been talking? I can't tell if I'm saying things out loud or if everything is all in my mind.

I vomited violently all over myself.

Defeated and desperate, worried that I was drifting in and out of consciousness, I whispered, "Brian, I have to go back to the hospital."

Gale's right. I am sick and I need help and I need someone who is a professional to take care of me.

"Okay," Brian replied, simply. He began gathering my things. Although he didn't say it, I'm sure he was also worried about surviving another night like we had experienced on Monday.

"Brian, grab water. Ensure. Socks. Towel." I rose from the sofa and made my way to the door, leaning on pieces of furniture as I passed: the bookcase to the chair, the chair to the bed. I sat on the bed, picked up a dirty shirt and pair of pants from the floor, and got dressed.

Brian instructed, "I'll go pull the car around and tell Sean and the girls to shut themselves up in another room." He ran down the stairs, holding my backpack. I picked up my Hillsborough Hospital mug from the nightstand and noticed my Bible next to it.

I need that for sure.

I shuffled out the door, retrieving my black coat from the hook as I passed it on the way to the stairs. Holding my Bible, mug, and coat, I slid down the steps on my butt as I had done two days earlier. Again, Brian helped guide me through the house to the car. As Brian started the car, I realized I was still wearing my Hillsborough Hospital bracelet from Monday on my wrist.

Maybe I'll get a new bracelet to add to the collection. Time to storm the hospital, take #2!

Having a plan of action made me feel a bit like my old self. I was always storming into action in one way or another—until that first night in Tampa.

16
Something Is Wrong

Tuesday, March 17

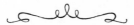

I began stirring by eight on Tuesday morning, and I knew Brian was awake too. "Brian, what time do we need to leave the apartment today? I want to clean the place before we leave. It's such a wreck right now. You know I always like to clean before I leave to go somewhere."

"We can take the PATH to Newark Penn Station and then take a sixteen-dollar short cab ride. So to be safe, let's leave at eleven to have plenty of time."

"Sounds good to me." I chuckled. "I swear we're the kings of saving money when it comes to getting to airports."

Trying not to wake the girls on the pullout couch in the living room, I tiptoed to the front door and retrieved our newspaper, then tiptoed back to the bedroom. I slid back into bed next to Brian and opened the paper.

"Brian, New York recorded 814 new cases of the virus yesterday. That's a big spike. Here's a quote from Mayor de Blasio: 'It's unbelievable how rapidly this crisis is growing. He says he expects as many as 10,000 cases in the city by next week."

Brian, still half-asleep, groaned and said, "Ugh, this is bad. I'm so glad we're leaving. It's clear this thing is out of control—it's beyond manageable at this point. Just need to get the girls out of here."

Nodding, I began reading an article about tourism in the city:

Major hotel chains are closing en masse, for the first time in history, because of the coronavirus—prompting requests for aid from President Trump. The New York Hilton Midtown on Sixth Avenue—the Big Apple's largest hotel—closed yesterday ... the city is likely to lose as many as 500,000 jobs in businesses that cater to tourists and people moving about the city. ... In one month, their lost wages amount to $1 billion.

Huh. I know the Marriott Vacation Club was still open yesterday. Wonder what's going to happen to it. And what's going to happen to my fellow tour guides? I hope everyone can make it financially through this craziness!

I shifted my attention to another article, this one listing all the new restrictions in the city. "We are getting out just in time, Brian. The city is shutting all nonessential businesses. I guess that means only police and fire departments, hospitals, grocery stores, and pharmacies can be open. Maybe gas stations, banks, and laundromats too. Also, starting today, gatherings of fifty or more people are banned. Last week you could have up to five hundred people!"

"It's the new normal—at least for a while." Brian sighed.

I set the paper aside so I would have something to read on the plane and grabbed my laptop off the nightstand. Scrolling through Facebook, I stopped to read an article on "what the coronavirus does to the body."

The course a patient's coronavirus will take is not yet fully understood. Some patients can remain stable for over a week and then suddenly develop pneumonia. Some patients seem to recover but then develop symptoms again. Some stay sick for weeks. Experts say that when patients recover, it is often because the supportive care—fluids, breathing support, and other treatment—allows them to outlast the worst effects of the inflammation caused by the virus.

It's clear this virus attacks people in different ways. The goal is not to get it to find out how it's gonna attack you!

I waited till nine to wake the girls, who were still comatose. "Time to get up," I said, turning on the lights. "We need to leave in about two hours."

I threw a load of laundry into the washer while the girls slowly got moving.

"If you two get dressed and packed in time, you could do a run to Starbucks," I suggested, hoping they could fill the time before we left with something they enjoyed. Also, sending them on a coffee run would get them out from underfoot, allowing me to concentrate on a deep clean of the apartment. A few minutes later, they were out the door to order their lattes at the Starbucks across the street.

We were all packed and ready to go by eleven. The pullout bed had been folded back into the couch, the rugs were vacuumed, and the floors swept clean of hair from three women. The bathroom was spotless, and the laundry was done—I threw the still-wet sheets from the girls' pullout bed over the bedroom and bathroom doors, as is my habit when I don't have time to babysit the dryer. I took one last look at our sweet, small apartment and said aloud, "See you in a few weeks!"

As we headed toward the front door, Brian pointed out the window and said, "Look outside; it's drizzling. Let's all grab an umbrella, and go ahead and put on our masks and gloves."

As I picked up an umbrella from the red bucket next to the door, I noticed my knee-length black wool coat hanging off the back of a chair at the living room table. I grabbed it and joined the group standing in the hallway. Noticing Brian's quizzical look, I said sheepishly, "I know, I know—I'm going to regret bringing this coat. I'll probably end up dragging it all over Florida! But I hate being cold on the plane, and it'll be cold getting to the airport too."

He shrugged and flashed me a "whatever" look.

After our PATH and cab trek, we arrived at Newark airport and stepped inside a barely recognizable Terminal C. "Wow, where is everybody?" Brian said aloud.

The ticketing area, normally bustling with activity and long lines, was almost bare. Only a few people stood in front of ticket agents, and no one seemed to be in a hurry—the first time I had ever witnessed that scene at one of the busiest airports in the country. We checked the girls' luggage, breezed through security, and found our gate with plenty of time to spare. In another surprise, we were among the first to board. Wading down the aisle to the middle of the plane, Brian and I located our seats and stashed my backpack and his carry-on in the overhead bin. I sat with the two girls in a row of three, while Brian sat directly opposite us on the other side of the aisle. I kept looking toward the door of the plane, waiting for the crush of passengers.

Is everyone just late today? Maybe they are coming at the last moment, in order to limit the amount of exposure inside the airport.

Fifteen minutes passed; few people boarded. Three rows in front of us and two rows behind us were completely empty. "Wow, Brian, I've never seen a plane so empty," I whispered, leaning across the aisle.

A plane built for 156 passengers held about thirty when the flight attendant announced, "This is the final boarding. If you'd like to put some distance between yourself and other passengers, you can. This is not a full flight."

At that announcement, the thirty passengers began dispersing throughout the plane, creating a few rows of distance between most passengers.

Brian leaned over and asked, "Y'all want to do the same? Christina, why don't you replace me so you can be alone in this row, and I'll move to the empty row behind."

Brian and I shifted seats, but the girls stayed put.

"We'll stay where we're at," said Mae from her window seat.

The lack of passengers had unnerved me, but I was heartened by the flight attendants as they walked up and down the aisle during the emergency instructions. They seemed carefree and relaxed—even jovial.

Whew, that makes me more comfortable. They don't seem in the least bit nervous. It's business as usual. Then the risk must be low.

I met Janelle's eyes and gave her a big smile. She returned it.

We're off to Florida. Off to my beloved home state. Off to another adventure! OUT of the drama that is New York City right now!

I drifted off to sleep quickly, exhausted from the morning's activities, and slept the entire way, waking only when the plane began to descend.

"Hey, Sean!" Brian yelled, as he spotted his brother alongside the curb in front of baggage claim.

Sean gave his girls a quick hug, then moved to the back and opened the trunk. "Did you all have a good time?" he asked.

I settled into the back seat with the girls while Brian climbed in next to his look-alike brother. Pulling out of the terminal, Sean announced, "We are going to Publix to get some steaks for tonight. We're celebrating you guys escaping New York!"

We all cheered, especially Brian. I knew he was really looking forward to spending some quality time with his brother.

They're going to have so much fun catching up, and so much fun drinking good wine and craft beer! And I'm sure Sean will like having us here to keep him company. He must be so lonely since Michelle's deployment.

On the drive to the grocery store I checked my cell phone. There was a text from Eddie, a teacher in California, who often brought groups to New York City. I had been leading tours for his groups for years.

"Hey Christina! My group is supposed to come to New York City in late June and of course you're our tour guide, but everyone wants to cancel because of the pandemic. But I tell them it's way too early for that. Don't you think?"

I texted back: "Yes, it's three months away! I think this will all blow over by then. I can't tell you what to do, but that does seem extreme. BTW, I'm in Florida for a mini-vacation. Love keeping up with you on Facebook! See you and the group hopefully in June!"

"Love keeping up with you too!" Eddie texted back. "Talk to you soon!"

In the grocery store parking lot, we saw a few people loading up their cars with what looked like enough groceries to last for weeks, but others seemed to be simply picking up a few items, like we were. Everyone appeared relaxed. Normal. I saw only three people wearing masks. No one looked worried about an impending viral storm. Did they have any idea how the fear of it was shutting down one of America's most important cities?

I remember this. Right after 9/11 it was the same way. New York was mired in grief, mourning, and shock, but when we traveled to Florida a few months after the attacks, it was total normalcy. New York City—always living in its own little bubble.

As we made our way to the store entrance, Brian advised, "Let's put on our masks, you all."

The girls and I pulled our masks from our purses, but Sean said, "I haven't been wearing one. Not many people are wearing them down here."

But Brian was firm. "We've all gotten into the habit of wearing them, Sean. I have an extra one for you!"

Sean took it and snickered, but he put it on.

At the entrance, we stood in a short line to get "sanitized towelettes." When it was my turn, I couldn't seem to separate the perforated sheets. A woman behind me looked impatient, so I used two hands to rip it off, touching a bit of the next sheet.

I think that just defeated the purpose.

Sean said, "I'll get the steaks; the rest of you get some sides. Meetcha in fifteen at the front!"

"Brian, I'm going down this aisle to get some kombucha!" I chirped, happy to stock up on my favorite drink and happy to be in sunny, carefree Florida. As I grabbed some large bottles of kombucha from a refrigerated display, I spotted a new-to-me drink.

Hard kombucha?! I've heard of such a product but have never seen it! Woohooo, I'm gonna get it!

Practically giddy, I checked out and joined the group at the entrance.

As we drove to Sean's home, Janelle asked, "Have you ever seen the show *Love Is Blind*?"

"No," I said. "Never heard of it. Is it good?"

"Yes, it's so much fun to watch. It's awesome. We could watch it tonight—what do you think?"

"It's a plan!!" I said as we pulled into the driveway.

Compared to our tiny New York apartment, Sean's 3,000-square-foot home seemed palatial. The two-story stucco house was only five years old, and still looked brand new. I stowed my backpack in the upstairs guest bedroom and then bounded down the stairs to find my hard kombucha. I settled into a massive, comfy couch in the kitchen/living room space and began sipping my delectable drink as I watched the guys grill and cook.

I love it when the Stanton boys take over the cooking. Their mom trained them well!

As I drank and lounged, I became aware of a tightness in my throat.

Must be this kombucha. I love it, but it does have a bitter taste.

Although I was eager for dinner, I was disappointed when my steak and asparagus and potatoes tasted bland.

I'm not about to tell the guys that these dishes need some seasoning, but boy—there's almost no flavor here at all.

I smiled as the girls told Sean about our New York City adventures, happy to know that despite the weirdness and drama, they had found the experience interesting. I was grateful that we had been able to spend some real quality time together.

"Okay! Let's watch *Love Is Blind*!" Janelle announced when dinner was over and the dishes were done.

"Woohooo!" I yelled, matching her excitement.

As Janelle searched for an episode, Brian sat down beside me and whispered, "Hey, I just checked the online news. One hundred new cases of the virus were counted in New York City today."

"Wow!" I whispered back. "In one *day*?!"

Brian nodded. "News reports say as of tonight, 108 people in the country have died of COVID."

The numbers were hard to comprehend.

I just really thought our government would contain it before it got to this point. How did this get so out of hand?

I tried to focus on the show, which was really fun. But as we watched, the tightness in my throat grew to an all-out sore throat.

Huh. Need to take some ibuprofen to beat that down. I'll bet Sean has some.

Although it was only 8:30 p.m., fatigue was settling over me like a heavy cloud. I rarely nod off while watching TV, but I slumped down into the couch and napped, waking when I felt Sean lay a quilt over me.

"Let's go upstairs and go to sleep, Christina," Brian said, touching my arm. I looked at the clock: 10:30. Had I been asleep for two hours?

I blinked my eyes, which were stinging and watery. It reminded me how my eyes felt after I swam open-eyed in a chlorine pool as a kid.

I gingerly rose from the couch and discovered that my body ached as if I had been battered. I stumbled to the staircase and had to use the railing to pull myself up each step.

Uh-oh, what's this? Why do I feel like I've been run over?

My throat was tight, and it hurt when I swallowed. When I fell into the bed, I felt super hot. "Brian, will you turn on the ceiling fan? I am hot, hot, hot!"

"Really?" he asked. "I'm not at all."

Brian is usually very sensitive to temperature and easily gets too hot or cold, but I rarely notice until it's an extreme. And now, it seemed extremely hot. Although I didn't want to go back downstairs, I realized I was very thirsty, so I dragged myself back to the kitchen to fill a glass of water. The trip seemed like a huge chore, as if I had aged twenty years in the last three hours.

Back in bed, I tossed and turned for hours, unable to get comfortable, when normally I fall asleep as soon as my head hits the pillow.

Something is wrong. Something is way wrong. I have never felt like this before. What is going on with my body?

17

HOSPITAL, TAKE #2

Wednesday, March 25, Evening

No tears flowed down my cheeks during our drive to the hospital this time, but I felt as if I were floating outside my body instead of inhabiting it.

"I'm sorry, Christina—sorry this is taking so long," Brian said, so worried he was shaking. "Looks like there's a lot more traffic at five in the afternoon than in the morning. The GPS says it will take an hour."

I slumped against the door, resigned. Suddenly, I sat up and yelled, "Where is the towel?"

"Right here!" Brian reached behind him and flung the towel over onto my lap. I quickly lifted it to my mouth and threw up, and then held the towel to my face in case it happened again.

"Brian … try again to get yourself a COVID test … at the hospital."

"The last time I was there they told me no, and I don't have any more symptoms now than I did then," he responded, obviously frustrated by the memory.

"But," I persisted as best I could, "you tell them … wife has it … they'll do it."

"No," Brian insisted. "I was told on the phone when I called Teladoc that there's no reason for me to take the test because if you have it, then I probably have it, so it's a moot point."

"But for proof ... it's important ... to be counted." I gave the argument one last try.

Brian remained silent as we drove up the now-familiar ramp and pulled into the emergency room lane. I pressed the window button with one finger and adjusted my mask with the other hand, trying to carefully fold the towel across my lap so that it would not leak its contents.

Leaning across me, Brian yelled out the window at the approaching attendant, "We're COVID-positive, and my wife needs help. This is the second time she's needed to go to the hospital."

The attendant halted a few feet away and yelled back, "Okay, gotcha. Where did she go before?"

I held up my wrist with the hospital tag as Brian and I both yelled, "Here!" She turned to retrieve a wheelchair while I slowly got out of the car. Brian came around and set the backpack on my lap while I nestled into the wheelchair. "She's been throwing up," Brian said to the attendant now behind me. "Should I get the towel in our car in case she throws up in the wheelchair?"

"No! Keep it in the car!"

"Bye, Christina! I love you!" Brian said sadly, waving as he stood outside the car. The attendant was backing me in through the hospital doors, and I kept my eyes locked on Brian's until the doors closed in front of me. I wondered when I'd see him again and what state I would be in by then. I felt like I was teetering on the edge of a steep precipice, and I couldn't see the bottom. The doors closed, and I was wheeled down the same employees-only route as I had traveled two days earlier, and we stopped outside my former room.

"Is there a room available?" my attendant asked a guy in scrubs who was walking past.

"No—all filled up," he said apathetically, and kept walking.

Without a word, my aide pushed on. Finally, she stopped and backed me into a large room, wheeling me next to the bed. "Okay, we're going to put you in here for the time being. Can you get into the bed on your own?"

"Yes," I said, placing my mug, backpack, coat, and Bible on the bed before slowly transferring myself. As I climbed into the bed, someone in scrubs approached my door and taped a piece of paper over the window, obscuring my view of any activity in the hall. I couldn't read the sign, but I could see a big red circle on the paper with a diagonal line across it.

Wow. "Warning! Dangerous Person Inside." I'm sure that's what the sign says—more or less. It's so wild that I'm the one to be scared of. Don't come near me, people!

"I'm going to cut your old tag off," my attendant said. "We're going to make a new one. And the information on this one will be helpful." She cut the tag off and left the room, dragging the wheelchair behind her. I looked around the room and noticed the clock: 6:15 p.m. Although I had been reluctant to return to the hospital, I was glad to be here. On my last visit, the IV fluids had made such a difference so quickly. I was actually eager to get one started this time.

I decided to settle in and get organized before I got the IV, since I knew the tubes and cords would restrict my movement. Unpacking my backpack, I set my bottles of water within easy reach, plugged in my cell phone and computer, and put on warm socks. Afterwards, I visited the toilet. I saw a hospital gown lying at the foot of the bed and decided to put it on.

Probably easier to pee if I don't have to get in and out of pants.

I rolled up my clothes and stuffed them into my backpack. Returning to the bed, I draped the blanket and my coat over me to stay warm.

I know the score now—this ain't my first time at the rodeo!

While I was unpacking, I kept glancing at the clock, expecting a nurse to be in at any time to talk to me about my symptoms, check my vital signs, discuss my medical history—all the things you expect when arriving at a hospital. As the minutes dragged on with no sign of *anyone*, I felt my anxiety climb higher and higher, even as I tried to reassure myself that I would feel better as soon as the IV got started.

My head was pounding, and mounting rumblings in my abdomen made me fear I would begin vomiting at any moment. Lifting the straw of my mug to my lips, I tried to focus on hydrating myself. Two refills later, I was still alone. I checked the clock: 7:30 p.m. Dialing the nurses' station from the hospital phone, I gasped, "Can someone come in ... and give me an IV? I need it. I need someone ... to help me!" This was worse than being at Sean's house—at least there, I had Brian to help me.

"Someone will come and help you soon," the woman on the end of the line assured.

Ten more minutes passed before a man and woman decked out in personal protective gear finally entered my room. "Hello, Christina. I understand you were recently admitted and have returned?" asked the man, skipping any introductions.

Should I ask their names? Nah, I so rarely see the same people twice. I can't remember all those people's names anyway. But it sure would be nice to know if I'm talking to a doctor or nurse or an admissions clerk.

"Yes, I was just here ... because ... I had low blood pressure issues ... I'm COVID-positive." I tried to be polite but insistent, mustering my strength to explain myself as best I could. "But ... Monday night ... I threw up ... had diarrhea ... had a 103 temperature all night. Ever since, I haven't been great."

As I croaked out my story, the woman snapped a new ID bracelet on my wrist.

"Okay, we're going to do a few tests, so just relax," the man said.

The female must have been a nurse because she took my blood pressure and taped a Pulse Oximeter to my middle finger. The male began taping multiple sensors onto my torso so they could test my heart rate. I lay back on the bed and sighed, relieved.

I'm going to get the help I need. They're going to get me better. Thank you, Lord, for this help! Thank you for bringing me here! This is exactly where I need to be.

The nurse reported, "Your blood pressure is fine, but your heart rate is very high, which is probably because you're dehydrated. We'll do an IV."

YES! That's what I'm here for! BRING IT!

The male asked, "What medicine have you been taking?"

I replied, "Only Tylenol and hydroxychloroquine ... but I haven't taken ... hydroxychloroquine since Monday night ... because of ... rash on my back. I'm not sure, but I'm wondering ... if hydroxychloroquine ... also caused ... some heart palpitations and swelling in my lips."

"Let me see it," he said, as he lifted me upright from my

pillow and manually leaned me forward. I felt a gloved hand move up and down my back. "No, you can't take that anymore," he said matter-of-factly, as he brought my gown back down and raised his stethoscope. He didn't address my mention of heart palpitations. "Do you have a cough?"

"I cough more and more ... but still not bad. Mucus ... or something ... has developed the last few days."

"Let me listen to your lungs." At his direction, I breathed in and out while he moved the stethoscope over my chest. "I hear some crackles—they are a lung sound indicative of fluid in your lungs. Okay, we'll be doing some more tests. She'll take care of your IV—I'll be back soon."

Crackles? Sounds like something good to eat, but what an awful word to describe health stuff.

"Hmmm," said the nurse, examining both of my arms. "We really can't use the vein they used on you before because it's still healing, and your vein in your antecubital doesn't look good in your other arm."

I cringed. Even though I was eager for the IV, I wasn't looking forward to the needle. The nurse kept tapping her fingers on different veins in both arms, then took my hands and turned them back and forth, examining them thoroughly as she decided what to do. She put a tight rubber band around my forearm, and I watched the vein fill with blood and deepen in color inside my elbow.

"I think we can actually use this one," she stated, before finally inserting the needle through the main vein in my forearm.

She warned, "This is inserted at a weird angle, so you'll have to hold your arm out in this direction to make sure the needle has access." She held my arm out to the side to demonstrate a palm-forward, ninety-degree angle. It seemed awkward.

"How will I use the bathroom?"

"I was going to suggest a bedpan," she replied. She picked up the hospital phone and asked, "Can someone hand in a bedpan?" Someone approached the door and cracked it open. A bedpan emerged through the crack, and the nurse walked to the door and retrieved it, clutching one corner. She returned and placed what looked like a pink dustpan into my hand. "Okay, here you go. You are *really* dehydrated, by the way." She walked to the sink, removed her gloves, and tossed them into the trash can.

I wasn't surprised. I wanted to tell the nurse that I had been drinking constantly, but I didn't have the energy. But even as she left the room, I started to feel the effects of the IV. My headache disappeared, the pressure in my chest eased, I felt like I could speak in full sentences again without wheezing, and I no longer felt like vomiting. I fell asleep, waking about a half hour later when I needed to use the bathroom. I moved my legs over the bed rail, trying to maintain my IV'd arm in the same erect position and balance the pan under my gown with the hand that was hooked up to the blood pressure monitor.

When I completed my business, I set the container on the floor and slid it under my bed. I hoped a nurse would empty it when it got full; I did not think I could balance the pan and maneuver myself to the bathroom while I was all hooked up.

I had just managed to hoist myself back onto the bed when the nurse returned. She checked my monitors and said, "Well, your heart rate is stabilized. We have a lot of tests we're going to do, just so you know. I'm going to take blood samples now, but the good news is I can do that from your IV needle, rather than tapping into another vein."

Thank you, Jesus, for this small mercy!

"We're also going to do a chest X-ray. And we'll see if your electrolytes are low through a urine sample."

I was grateful to hear that there was an action plan and heartened to feel like the medical personnel were taking me seriously. A succession of people subsequently came in to perform the tests—I saw twice as many people in an hour as I had seen during my entire previous hospital visit.

Abruptly, another nurse came in and announced, "We're going to keep you overnight, so we're moving you to a different room, okay?" She picked up my backpack from the floor and moved it to my outstretched hands.

"Oh—okay," I stammered. Grabbing the items I'd positioned around me for easy access, I threw them into the backpack as quickly as possible, since the nurse seemed to be in a hurry. A wheelchair emerged, and I gingerly maneuvered my way around multiple tubes and wires to the chair. After I was unhooked from the machines, I was rolled down the hall with my IV in tow back to the hospital area where I had been Sunday night.

I was soon installed in a similar room, which included one bed, a small window and TV, a toilet and sink inside the main room, and that special anteroom that separated me from the hall. This seemed more dignified somehow than having a hand-drawn sign on my door warning others away from me.

I nestled in, feeling taken care of and thoroughly attended to. I felt certain that being here would give me the help I needed to emerge from this sickness post-haste, put this misery behind me, and return to my family. It had to end soon, didn't it? I had been sick for so long! It had been nine days since I had fallen asleep on Sean's couch while we were watching TV. Nine days since I had tossed and turned, wondering what was going wrong with my body. Looking back now, I could see that's where this had started, and I had been sliding downhill ever since.

18

Isolated on My "Mini-Vacation"

Friday, March 20

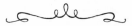

I woke at eight, like normal, but nothing else seemed normal. I blinked and gazed around the unfamiliar room, and it took me a minute to remember where I was. It had been another uncomfortable night, filled with tossing and turning and drinking water and Gatorade and peeing it right out. I sat up on the bed and reached for my plastic bottle of water, beginning another day of battling in vain to soothe my parched throat.

My phone told me it was Friday. If my phone was right, I was entering my third day alone in this room. I had chosen to hunker down here Wednesday morning; I didn't know what was ailing me, but I worried that I might be contagious. Brian had been sleeping on the small sofa in the nearby family room, not the ideal arrangement for my six-foot, two-hundred-pound husband. I knew he wasn't getting much sleep because he woke every time I headed to the bathroom down the hall—and I made that trip many times every night.

Slowly and gingerly, I rose from the bed and wobbled to the bathroom to take a shower. As I began my daily ritual of conditioning my hair, my knees began to buckle and the bathroom began to spin. Panicking, I lowered myself into a seated position on the floor of the tub and spread out my legs in front of me. The room felt very hot and steamy, so with my right foot, I nudged the faucet toward colder water. Pulling back the shower curtain, I leaned over the edge of the tub, desperate for some fresh air.

I sat there for a full ten minutes, splayed out in the tub, cold water flowing over my body, which was half in and half out of the tub. Gradually, the room stopped spinning, and I finally felt brave enough to stand up and attempt a dash back to the bedroom. Grabbing a towel as I stumbled out of the bathroom, I wrapped it around my very wet body and made a beeline for the bed.

Brian witnessed this frantic crossing, and he followed me as I dove into the bed, dripping and shaking.

"What's wrong, Christina?"

"I almost fainted in the shower!"

"I'm going to call Teladoc and see if we can get help for you." Brian grabbed the computer and sat down on the other side of the bed. I tried to remain still and regroup.

"Okay, I found someone to call, and they're telling me I can have an appointment in an hour."

"Great. Thanks." I had gotten into the habit of speaking only in short sentences the past few days, as I always felt out of breath.

At 10 a.m., Brian dialed the doctor. "I'll speak for you," he told me, "but I will put the doctor on speaker phone so you can hear what she's saying."

"Thanks, Brian," I murmured.

"Hello, my name is Brian Stanton and I'm calling on behalf of my wife, who isn't feeling well. She feels winded, achy, she runs a fever once or twice a day, and has lost her sense of taste and smell, among other symptoms. We live in New York City, but just arrived here Tuesday. We don't know if she has the coronavirus or not, but she's rarely sick. I was wondering if you could prescribe anything?"

I was dismayed by the doctor's reply. "If you are just arriving from New York City, you wouldn't be used to Central Florida during pollen season. Don't underestimate how pollen can affect the body. Many people have an adverse immune response when they breathe in pollen. In people with pollen allergies, the immune system mistakenly identifies the harmless pollen as a dangerous intruder. It begins to produce chemicals to fight against the pollen. This is known as an allergic reaction, and a lot of the symptoms you're describing sound like a reaction to pollen."

"Oh, okay," Brian said, hesitating. "But what if it's COVID? Should we try to get a test?"

"At this point, you need to call the CDC to get information for testing sites," she said. "We don't know where to refer you, and we don't offer testing. I can prescribe benzonatate if you develop a cough. And a Z-Pak might be good as well. What is your local CVS pharmacy so I can call this in?"

Brian looked up the address and CVS phone number and gave it to her. "Thank you, ma'am, I'm hoping this is it. It's a relief to know this might be allergy-related."

"Well, that's interesting!" Brian said, hanging up and turning to face me. "Pollen. I would never have guessed that could be a cause of your symptoms."

"Brian, I'm from Florida," I said weakly. I paused and then continued, my voice growing stronger as my frustration rose.

"I grew up in a pollen epicenter! This isn't a pollen allergy situation!"

"Well, at least we can get some drugs that might make you feel better," Brian said, picking up the phone to call the pharmacy.

"Hi, this is Brian Stanton. Have you received a prescription for me?" Brian again put the phone on speaker.

"I'm sorry, but nobody has this pill—there's been such a high demand for benzonatate that it's sold out everywhere and I have no estimated date of when we'll get it in. But we have the Z-Pak. You can come pick that up anytime. Use the drive-through."

"Christina, I'm off to the CVS drive-through. I'll be back!"

"Brian, before you go, I want to know—are you feeling okay?"

"Well," he answered reluctantly, "I actually felt like I might have had a fever when I woke up this morning. But by the time I got my act together to take my temperature, it had gone away. Also, my stomach is gurgling. It's a strange sound. It's weird. I can't make sense of it. I don't know why it's doing that."

"What about the girls and Sean?" I asked, apprehensively.

"Oh, they're fine. Everyone else seems fine."

Good. Whatever I have hasn't spread to the girls. I hope I haven't given anything to Brian.

Brian left, and I got up and settled onto the sofa. Feeling lonely, I picked up my computer, wanting to give my girlfriends an update. I wrote a message in a group chat that includes four of my best girlfriends from childhood, who are scattered throughout the country.

"Hi Ladies, I left NYC and am now with Brian's family near Tampa. I've been feeling bad the last few days. I'm worried I have the virus. Just feel crummy."

Their responses came back quickly.

"Why are you in Florida?"

"Are you sure it's the virus? It's probably the flu—I hear they're very similar!"

"Well, if you think you have it, go get tested! ASAP!"

I stared at my phone dumbfounded. Their reactions made me realize the chasm between us. In New York City, the virus was front and center and on everyone's mind. But where my friends lived, they weren't watching the number of infected people rise daily while the number of available hospital beds dwindled. The virus wasn't dominating every bit of news or every aspect of their daily lives like it was for people in New York.

The fact that they thought it was easy to get a COVID test reminded me of the misinformation out there. I had tried twice to get a test, but even health professionals didn't know where I could get one. It was apparent my friends didn't understand the severity of the outbreak in New York City, or that it was a real possibility I had contracted the virus. They were certainly concerned about my welfare but not concerned that I was facing something potentially so dire.

Their reactions reminded me of what happened after 9/11. My friends outside of New York were horrified by the attacks, but their lives were not totally upended like mine was. I remember feeling broken and alone in the aftermath, while my friends continued their daily routines. Trying to hide my disappointment, I bade a pleasant farewell and got off the chat.

I wondered if I should contact my mother. Should I tell Mom I'm sick? I decided against it.

I don't even know what sickness I have, and she would worry. Maybe I should just go to Tallahassee when I get better and surprise her! That would be fun!

As the day went on, I continued switching from bed to sofa, interrupted by frequent trips to the bathroom. I hit the bed when I felt sleepy, but I rarely actually slept. The sofa was my preferred location when I wanted to read the news or check my email or attempt to read a book.

The one window in the room looked out over the beautiful backyard. Sometimes I would stare outside the window and enjoy the sunlight on my face while I watched my nieces sit at the picnic table under the tall oak trees or in the Adirondack chairs circled around the stone firepit. I liked watching them from the window, yet it made me wistful because I couldn't join them.

Soon, soon. I just need to get over whatever this is so I can go and hang out with them. I really miss our talks.

I was resting in bed at five in the afternoon when I felt my face flush and grow hot.

I think my temperature is spiking. Wow, I can't get used to these high fevers. I don't remember having a temperature like this since I was a kid. What a yucky sensation.

I rose from the bed, headed over to my nest of necessities, and downed a couple of Tylenol. I turned to walk to the bathroom but stumbled, feeling lightheaded and weak. Realizing it would be at least twenty more steps until I made it to the bathroom, I sank back down on the bed.

Brian knocked on the door and then poked his head in.

"Christina, I just wanted to check in on you. Is everything okay?"

"I'm worried I'm not gonna be able to make it to the bathroom. Can you ask your brother if he has a bucket?"

"Are you serious, Christina? C'mon! You don't need a bucket!"

"I do, Brian. I'm serious. I have to get up every fifteen minutes or so, and it's just getting harder and harder to do that. I keep worrying I won't make it all the way to the bathroom!"

"Okay, I'll go down and ask. But I hope you're exaggerating!"

Brian returned soon with a white five-gallon bucket. "Sean says this is the bucket he uses when he makes homemade ice cream. Only use this if you *really* need it, okay?"

He strategically set the bucket on the floor between the sofa and the bed.

"Sorry, Brian, I've got to use the bucket right now." As I rushed to the bucket, Brian fled the room, horrified.

Well, that's the last time poor Sean will use this bucket to make homemade ice cream.

Afterward, I returned to the bed. When I lay flat and still, I felt fine. It was moving that threw everything out of whack.

Another knock on the door.

"Christina, your dinner is outside on the floor!" Brian yelled. For the past couple of days, he had been delivering my meals and supplies outside the door to minimize contact. I wasn't hungry at all, but I walked across the room, opened the door, and retrieved the tray. I shut the door with my foot and moved the tray to the side of the bed.

Climbing back into bed, I propped myself up on a pillow and transferred the tray onto my belly.

Angel-hair pasta in a garlic sauce with vegetables. One of Sean's concoctions, obviously! Sean is such a good cook. I sure wish I could taste this pasta. Or at least smell it!

I twirled the pasta around my fork, but as I brought the food close to my mouth, I recoiled, trying to suppress the bile that rose suddenly in my throat. I threw the fork back on the plate and shoved the tray to the bed as I concentrated on quelling my nausea.

What was that? I almost never throw up. I don't think I've thrown up since that night I drank too much at that crazy party. But that was twenty-plus years ago.

I remained still, hoping the nausea would pass. I could hear the TV from the living room on the ground floor. Bursts of laughter and snippets of conversation from Brian, Sean, and the girls floated up the stairs.

Dangit, they're all having fun watching a movie and I'm stuck up here. I so wish I was down there to enjoy the family time with them!

When I felt more stable, I moved back to the sofa, opened my laptop, and clicked on Facebook. I considered writing a post informing my friends that I wasn't feeling well but decided against it as I scrolled through my newsfeed. I recognized a theme in various posts from friends and articles people were sharing: fear. Everyone was afraid of the future, but no one seemed to know what to do.

Nah—I'm certainly not going to mention I'm sick. I don't want anyone to worry, and I don't want to bring attention to myself.

Instead of writing, I decided to research the coronavirus, reading medical articles and first-person accounts, trying to educate myself about the virus and its symptoms. Most of the articles highlighted respiratory ailments and coughs. One woman described her COVID condition as akin to having "swallowed glass."

That sounds awful! I'm glad I don't feel like that! And I don't have a cough, so maybe I don't have the virus after all!

I ended up on the *New York Post* website and was alarmed to read the headline "Coronavirus killing more than one person per household."

Wow, according to this article, this morning's death toll was at twenty-nine, but the day is ending at forty-three.

The city's positive cases had climbed from 5,151 to 5,683 during the day. A major disaster declaration had been announced for New York over the coronavirus.

That usually only happens for natural disasters, like Hurricane Sandy. And Governor Cuomo has issued a statewide lockdown starting Sunday. Poor New York City! This is all looking so bad.

I looked away from the computer and concentrated on the muffled sounds of laughter and conversation emanating from downstairs.

Dear Lord, please heal me so I can get back to normal. Please don't let me have this coronavirus. Let me just have some flu, where I'll wake up tomorrow and be fine. I just want to enjoy this "mini-vacation" you blessed us with here in Florida.

I picked up my Gatorade and started chugging—again.

19

FIFTY/FIFTY

Wednesday, March 25, Night

I was only alone in the room for a few minutes before a nurse arrived to re-hook the heart monitor. Then she pulled a tray table alongside my bed and announced, "I'll be back in a moment with your dinner."

I was surprised that they would bring me dinner after 9 p.m., but I resolved to try to eat something even though I was not hungry. I knew I needed nutrition to regain my strength.

I slid my backpack up from the bottom of the bed and pulled out my computer, cell phone, and the hospital mug. I then unfolded the small blanket and stretched it across me before covering it lengthwise with my coat. I smiled weakly remembering how Brian had made fun of me bringing the wool coat to Florida. Lastly, I retrieved my Bible and set it on the rolling tray table. Placing my hand on its worn cover, I felt comforted to have something so familiar and important with me in this cold, lonely, and completely unfamiliar environment.

The nurse, accompanied by another woman whom I thought was a nurse, backed in with a tray of food as soon as I had gotten settled. "Here's your dinner: Salisbury steak and corn, with a container of fruit."

She didn't say anything about a low-sodium meal like the last time I was here. Does that mean anything, like, my heart rate is better?

The nurse said, "I want to introduce you to Judith, who is a representative from the CDC. She has a few things to ask you."

"Hi!" I said, picking at the corn.

Oh wow—a representative from the Centers for Disease Control and Prevention is here to talk to me! I feel so VIP.

"Hi, Christina," Judith said. "I just want to know about your story. How you recognized your symptoms and how you are today. I want to hear anything you want to tell me about your journey."

As Judith interviewed me, I hoped the information I was providing would be helpful. I knew I was one of the earlier cases—especially in this area—and I was aware the country was still in the early stages of developing a plan of attack against the virus.

I hope they are interviewing all of us! Collectively, all our stories could increase our knowledge of how to combat this terrible thing. Make it easier for the people getting sick after us!

"It sounds like you have a mild case. Well, thank you for this information, and I hope you get better soon!" Judith said politely after about ten minutes. She rose from her chair and began the exit ritual.

A "mild case"? I wonder what the differences are between mild, severe, and light? And who decides? Interesting she considers me "mild."

About 10 p.m., a diminutive male doctor with dark brown eyes, heavily protected with a mask, visor, and several layers of scrubs like everyone, entered and headed directly to the computer mounted on a shelf in the middle of the room.

"Hi, Christina, I'm Dr. Khan," he said in a soft voice, while pecking at the computer.

"Hello," I said, studying his silhouette reflected by the light of the computer.

He spent several moments studying the screen, then finally said, "I want to give you some updates. Christina, your heart is better, but the tests are showing you have some issues that will necessitate keeping you here for observation. Tests are showing you have dangerously high ferritin and lactate dehydrogenase, and dangerously low blood urea nitrogen levels. These have to do with issues involving your heart, liver, tissue damage, among other possibilities."

He continued in his gentle tone, "Christina, you have extra weight, which can give you an increased risk of severe illness from the coronavirus. And I read your report—you mentioned '9/11 lungs.' That pre-existing condition might have made you more vulnerable to the virus because your lungs are already damaged from the dust you inhaled in Lower Manhattan. Your constitution has and will continue to dictate how this plays out."

"Okayyyyyyy."

Hearing these strange medical terms and learning that my test results were abnormal filled me with anxiety. Was the virus attacking my organs? Would there be long-term damage? These questions led me down a terrifying road, and to the next question, which I was almost too afraid to ask.

"Doctor," I began, taking a deep breath. "I want to know something—I want you to be honest with me. Can you tell me what my chances are of surviving COVID?"

His eyes seemed to droop behind his visor, and he turned to face me, staring straight into my eyes.

"Christina, I think your chances of survival are fifty/fifty."

My breath stopped. "What? I have a fifty/fifty chance of making it through this? Why? Why me?"

I had demanded honesty, but I had not expected his response.

His lips continued to move, but either his voice trailed off or I simply could not hear him anymore. I could not digest any more bad news.

Was my life going to come down to a flip of the coin? Heads I live or tails I die?

I began to blame myself.

Why had I let myself gain so much weight!? I survived 9/11, but it's coming back to haunt me. I thought we were doing the right thing to leave the city—but it looks like we should have left YEARS ago!

"Get some rest, Christina. I'll come check on you tomorrow."

Dr. Khan walked to the trash can to begin the exit ritual I now knew so well.

My first thought was to call Brian immediately. I picked up the phone and unlocked it but stopped before I tapped "call."

What would I say? "Hi, the doctor just told me that me—your wife of twenty years—has a fifty/fifty chance of surviving COVID?"

I was still holding the phone, trying to figure out what to tell Brian, when it began to ring. The caller ID flashed "Unknown Caller." I almost didn't answer because I didn't want to deal with a creepy spam call on top of what I had just learned from the doctor. But spammers don't usually call at 10:30 p.m., and I didn't want to be alone with my thoughts, so I took a risk and answered.

"Hello?" I ventured cautiously.

"Hey, Christina, it's Pastor Dimas, calling from the Bronx! I just heard you're in the hospital and I want to pray for you. Sorry to call so late—I hope I didn't wake you."

"Pastor Dimas! My old friend! It's so good to hear from you!"

It was so nice to hear a familiar voice. I had met Pastor Dimas Salaberrios in 2002 at a new pastor training program through the Redeemer Church Planting Center, where I had a job as an assistant. He was hard to miss. The six-foot-five African-American man commanded attention whenever he walked into a room, and his charisma drew people from all walks of life toward him, especially after they learned how God had saved him from a life as a drug dealer and led him to become a pastor. In 2005 we became cofounders of a Thanksgiving meal event in the Bronx that still takes place each November.

"I'm back in the hospital, Pastor Dimas. I just talked to the doctor, and he said I have a fifty/fifty chance of dying from this thing." Tears began streaming down my cheeks as I spoke those words for the first time. "Please pray for me, Brian, and the family."

"Lord, please comfort Christina," Pastor Dimas began praying. "Please heal her, please heal her family. Lord, listen to your children crying out to you—hear our pain and suffering; you are the great comforter and healer. Heal this family, heal our nation, heal the world. You are sovereign, Lord; we ask in the name of the Holy Spirit to heal this world and alleviate the suffering from this plague, Father God ..."

Ending his prayer, Pastor Dimas said to me, "Christina, if you get to where you are too ill or too tired to pray, remember Romans 8:26–27, okay? Let me read that to you:

In the same way, the Spirit also comes to help us, weak as we are. For we do not know how we ought to pray; the Spirit himself pleads with God for us in groans that words cannot express. And God, who sees into our hearts, knows what the thought of the Spirit is; because the Spirit pleads with God on behalf of his people and in accordance with his will.

"The Holy Spirit will lift you up, Christina. And just know, so, so many people are praying for you. Girl, you are covered."

"Thank you *so* much, Pastor Dimas!" I said, full of gratitude. Hanging up the phone, I lay still for a while, just looking at the ceiling.

"Lord," I said aloud. "It's just you and me. If you intend for this to be the end of the road for me, Lord, if that's in your will, please accept me into your kingdom. Forgive my sins, forgive me for all the missed opportunities of proclaiming your name to others. Forgive me for anger and self-righteousness when I didn't get my way, forgive me for not trusting you fully and relying on myself. Thank you for a wonderful life, a wonderful husband, wonderful friends. I've been so blessed."

Then I pointed toward the ceiling and continued, "But, Lord, my request is that you let me live. My life is yours. I don't have any more professional goals or aspirations for myself. I just want a life that fulfills your purpose only. Please spare me, Lord."

I began to speak louder and louder.

"Spare me, but also put me to use. I know whether it's now or later, my life will end, but I request more time here. I'm not ready yet, Lord, not yet. I have more people to love, more people I want to help. I don't want to leave Brian. I want more of you on this earth before I meet you in heaven. But if you want to call me home, please prepare me. Lord, when Dad died, he was unprepared. He didn't want to go. He fought and was bitter that he was being called home. I don't want to do it that way. Teach me how to let go, if it's time for me to go to you. And please watch over Brian while he remains here. Thank you for giving me such a blessed life, thank you for the health of my nieces and Brian and Sean, Lord!"

I wondered if the nurses could hear me, or if my fervent prayers might pull out some cords of the IV or set off alarms. I decided I didn't care.

I'm having my talk with God. If they think I'm hallucinating, well, then, maybe they'll keep me "under observation" for longer. Lord, please give those nurses and doctors wisdom to deal with "my constitution," but Jesus—the rest is in your hands!

20

BACK HOME AGAIN

Thursday, March 26

I slept fitfully throughout the night, waking with a start when a nurse arrived about seven with my breakfast.

"Hello, good morning! I have breakfast for you—pancakes!" she chirped. "How are you feeling?

"I'm fine," I answered groggily.

As I emerged from my sleep, I looked around the room, at the nurse, and down at my body, covered in my coat and a thin sheet with my bright blue-socked feet poking out below the pseudo-coverings. I felt a sense of relief.

I'm still here. I'm still alive! Not today, satanic virus. One day at a time I'm gonna fight you, and I'm gonna fight hard. This is the day that the Lord has made; I will rejoice and be glad in it!

The nurse checked my temperature. "Ninety-eight!"

I smiled, relieved to hear a number that didn't start with a one. "Oh good," I said. "Will I be getting another IV?"

"I don't think so at this point. Your blood pressure and heart rate look good. Have you had any diarrhea?"

"No. No diarrhea or vomiting since I got the IV yesterday."

The nurse made all her usual checks of me and the monitors and then began the elaborate scrubbing ritual. "A doctor should be coming in soon to talk to you about next steps," she told me as she exited.

Hmmm. I certainly hope those next steps aren't right out the door to return home!

I ate as much of my breakfast as I could manage and then phoned Brian. "Hey, hon, how is everyone today?"

"I think everyone's okay—no news is good news," Brian replied. "I'm feeling good. How are you?"

"I'm feeling okay," I replied. "A whole lot better than when I got here." I mentioned the abnormal test findings Dr. Khan had told me about yesterday but didn't mention the doctor's fifty/fifty prognosis. I simply didn't know how to broach that topic.

"I don't know when or if they plan to make me go home today. I figure the longer I stay, the more of a fighting chance I have against the bugs. Remember your Teladoc doctor said he's noticed his COVID-positive patients are having symptoms for two weeks, and since my symptoms started on March 17, I'm on day ten. Maybe only four more days to go! Every day here in the hospital is one day closer to this being over. And I really believe that every day at the hospital gives me more strength to fight stronger at home."

"I agree, Christina," Brian reassured me. "Let me know how things go today. Call and give me updates whenever you can."

I hung up, feeling a little guilty that I had not shared the doctor's thoughts about my chances of survival. I didn't want Brian to worry or hear the fear in my voice. I had tried to sound positive and upbeat during our call, and I did maintain a will to fight and experienced bursts of optimism. But it could turn on a dime, and I'd feel worn out and discouraged. Even more alarming were the sustained, recurring trips into my own mind where it felt like my body was trying to force me to disconnect from my surroundings. This virus was relentless.

Wanting to stay focused, I decided to check my emails and social media. Picking up my laptop with my right hand, I maneuvered it to rest on my belly, realizing I would be doing little typing because the IV and other wires and leads were attached to all but four of my ten fingers. I scrolled through my many emails, mostly from friends inquiring about my health. I opened one from Edie, a friend from college who wanted to send me some vitamin C supplements. Her generosity cheered me up.

Praise you, Lord, for my college buds! They are SO coming through for me now!

One Facebook acquaintance asked, "Hey Christina, you indicate that your brother-in-law and nieces are positive. Are you sure? Have they taken the test?"

The message irritated me. No, they had not taken the test to find out if they had the novel coronavirus that causes COVID-19 because they couldn't find any doctor or hospital or government agency that would give them the test! But we were all living in the same house and all experiencing some of the same symptoms—even the doctors told them to assume they had COVID. Why were people questioning our conclusion? How could we possibly have a different one?

But then I began scrolling through my Facebook newsfeed and found article after article related to testing for the virus, or the lack of testing for the virus, and who was eligible to get tested, and whether COVID cases were being overreported or underreported. I was also surprised to find so many headlines about hydroxychloroquine and what President Trump had said or not said about the drug. I was surprised to see that so many of the articles seemed to be written from a political slant.

As I scrolled past headlines such as "Joe Biden Is Trying to Be Heard on the Virus. Can He Break Through?" and "Trump Has Given Unusual Leeway to Fauci, but Aides Say He's Losing His Patience," I sat back in frustration.

Why is COVID medicine tied up with politics? Seems like strange bedfellows. I'm no fan of hydroxychloroquine, but that's because of what happened to me. It has NOTHING to do with whether I'm a Republican or a Democrat! And why is anyone arguing about testing? It seems like you should be able to get a test if you want it or believe you're infected. I'm so glad I got tested, but sad I had to get super sick and be in the hospital to get it. And why can't Brian or Sean or Janelle or Mae get a test? It just helps to know exactly what we are battling!

It was easy to see that the arguments and debates were turning angry, although I wasn't sure why. I remembered how much fear and confusion had surrounded 9/11, even without forums like Facebook or Twitter. Social media was just intensifying and magnifying the confusion and so I decided that I should shut off all the "noise" today. I wanted to connect with people and read their words of encouragement, but I was getting sucked into all the anger and sadness swirling through my newsfeed. Time to disconnect for a while.

The door opened and a tall man entered—another new face. "Hi, Christina. I'm Dr. Erlinde. You're stabilized and looking better than when you came here yesterday."

Anxiety shot through me like an electric current, which intensified with his next words.

"We're going to send you on home. We'll send you off with some medication—not hydroxychloroquine because of your reaction to that—but other meds that will help you if you have any ancillary issues like a cough or nausea or diarrhea ..."

I cut him off, tears welling up in my eyes and my voice rising in panic. "Why are you sending me home? I've been here for less than twenty-four hours! I got here at six last night and it's 9:15 a.m. now! I was told I have a fifty/fifty chance of living yesterday! Won't the odds of me surviving this get better if I'm here getting monitored—you all fight this so much better than I can!"

He tried to calm me with a soothing tone, but his words just scared me more.

"Yes, there are lots of things that can go wrong when you leave the hospital—electrolyte imbalance, issues with your heart and liver, and based on the lab findings, you might have some long-term issues to deal with once this is over. But at this point, there's really nothing more we can do for you here."

I wasn't buying it and launched into a steady stream of objections, not sure if I was making much sense but feeling the need to be heard.

"I don't agree that there is *nothing* you can do for me; the IV hydration made a *huge* difference. It's been twice now that I've arrived at the hospital dehydrated. I'm in a house with four COVID-positive people, and I'm the sickest. Could I make them sicker with my presence? If so, that seems reason enough to keep me here! I understand that caring for someone who has the virus during the entire trajectory of the virus is *not* the goal of hospitals, but obviously I'm not battling a light case of this, and I've read that the virus can cause someone to take a turn for the worse at any moment. You can imagine I'd want to be *here* rather than at *home* when or if that happens!"

"Oh, I wasn't aware of your family," he said. His tone was emotionless and flat; clearly, my overwrought pleas were not making a difference. "You all just need to keep quarantining together and make sure you don't expose yourselves to anyone…"

I cut him off. "Well, of course we're not out and about. No one is going anywhere. Although that sure makes it hard for us to get the food and medicines we need. And it also makes it harder for any of them to take care of me! I need to be here where professionals can take care of me because my family should be saving their energy for their own fight."

He changed the subject. "What day do you think you're on in your fight with this?"

"Day ten."

"I think you'll have another week of this," he said, bluntly. "I know it's scary, but we've done all we can for you. Go home and do the best you can."

My heart sank.

A WEEK? Every day is torture—I can't imagine I'll be able to stand another week of this, if I even make it to a week! I feel like I'm not just fighting this virus, I'm fighting to get the hospital to help me fight it. Well, one thing's for sure, I'm keeping this bracelet on. And if I have to "hospital-storm" a third time, I will!

When the doctor left the room, I called Brian. "They're making me go home again."

Brian exhaled slowly. "Awww, I'm so sorry, Pea!"

"This feels like déjà vu—and is so frustrating! I feel so down right now. I can't handle another night like Monday."

"God's got this, Christina. I know it's frustrating, but we have to keep the faith. Just let me know when I can come get you. By the way, I called your mom and gave her an update on you. I know she wanted to know. And Stephanie's Gatorade arrived! She bought a truly massive amount of Gatorade for us."

"That's awesome! Thank you for calling Mom. I just wasn't up to that conversation. I don't want to leave here, but I'm looking forward to seeing you!"

Soon after, my phone rang, flashing a number I didn't recognize. The last time I answered an unknown caller, I had received a blessing from Pastor Dimas, so I decided to pick up again. "Hello?"

"Hi, Christina, this is Kathryn, and I represent the office of Samaritan's Purse. I know you're on our DART team, and I've heard you are sick from COVID. I'd like to pray with you and hear how Samaritan's Purse can pray for you in the days ahead."

"Oh, how kind! That's awesome, thank you."

I quickly updated Kathryn about me and my family, grateful that I had applied to work with Samaritan Purse's International Disaster Assistance Response Team a year ago. I had been hoping to be deployed overseas to help communities who had suffered through a natural or manmade disaster, but I'd not been able to take the minimum three weeks off to be on a team.

Maybe if I survive this, I'll finally have the time to go help. What a great thing to keep as a goal!

"Kathryn, I really, really wish I could know how this is all going to end. Like, I wish I could just fast-forward a month and know how all this plays out. Did I survive? I know this thing can go from mild to deadly in an instant—I've heard the tales. It's almost like I want to see into the future to know if

I'm still alive, so I can quit worrying now. I want to know now how my story ends."

"But that's what faith is for," Kathryn gently countered. "To have faith that God's got this, he knows the future, and he's in control."

My anxiety about leaving the hospital diminished as she spoke. "Thanks so much for that reminder—it's such a blessing you called. And hey, I have heard about the team en route to New York City—where you're going to set up tents in Central Park and have medical DART members help the overflowing hospitals. Bless you all! I wish I could get deployed to help, but obviously that's not going to happen this go-around."

"Well, concentrate on fighting so you can deploy with us and be a part of another team in the future," Kathryn said.

"That's an awesome thing to look forward to, thank you!"

Wow, God is just sending me all these wonderful assurances from unexpected people. Thank you, Lord!

My hospital phone rang not long after my call with Kathryn ended.

"Hello, Christina, it's Dr. Erlinde. You are free to go. A nurse will be bringing you some medicine: acetaminophen, benzonatate, and Tussin. These will treat your cough and fever. She'll include instructions and exit papers. Be well!"

I wasn't overly impressed with the offerings, especially because I had not had much of a cough.

I sure wish there was a pill called Covidbuhbye that actually addressed this virus!

But I was glad to be taking something home since none of us could visit a drugstore—and there was no guarantee of finding the medicine we needed even if we could get there.

It felt odd to be dismissed over the phone, but I was getting used to people avoiding contact with me as much as possible. Although I did not have my formal release, I texted Brian and asked him to come get me, knowing it would be forty minutes or more before he would arrive.

I really, really hope this is the last time at the hospital. Lord, please let this be the end of all of this!

While I waited for Brian, I wrote a CaringBridge post with "50/50" as the title, letting my friends know that I was again leaving the hospital and also informing them of my doctor's sobering outlook. I was careful not to check any emails or social media, remembering my vow to "shut off the noise" for a while.

Catching sight of Brian at the ER entrance gave me a jolt of energy and hope.

I need to be with Brian. He wouldn't ever leave my side; he'll do anything he can possibly do to keep me alive. But if things go in another direction, I can approach it with courage if he's with me. I wouldn't want to leave this earth without him near to pray for and with me, and send me off to rest in power!

We reached Sean's house about noon, and as Brian parked the car, I felt relief. There may be a battle ahead, but if I wasn't going to be fighting it in the hospital, this place was certainly the next best thing. I swung by the kitchen before heading upstairs and discovered a stack of Gatorade almost as tall as my waist sitting next to the fridge. The kindness of my friend touched my heart and literally made me feel better physically.

Lord, please bless Stephanie—thank you for showing your kindness through others such as her! It truly restores me in every sense of the word.

As I closed the fridge, I caught a glimpse of a can of hard kombucha I had bought on the day we arrived from New York. The sight of it now turned my stomach, and I realized that I was going to have to be very careful in the next few days. My choices and my actions could literally be the difference between life and death for me.

A text buzzed in. I looked at the screen and could see Tony Hale had uploaded a video. I pressed play, and the face of a young man I didn't recognize filled the screen. He boomed, "Hey, Mae and Janelle! It's Matty Cardarople from *Stranger Things* and *A Series of Unfortunate Events*! And my puppy Azoom!" The video zoomed in on a tiny Pomeranian, then back to the young man.

He spent ten minutes expressing apologies for this tough time and offering encouraging words and exhortations for staying positive and practicing self-care. Matthew had clearly spent a lot of time and effort to create a generous, kind, supportive, and very personal message for two strangers, my nieces.

I immediately texted Tony. "Look at what you did! Thank you SOO much!!!"

"Matthew's a friend, and he was happy to do it. I hope your nieces like it!"

I immediately forwarded Matthew's video to my nieces, and as I climbed the stairs to the bedroom, I could hear squeals of delight coming from their bedrooms.

I'm so thrilled Tony did that. How special it must have made Mae and Janelle feel! I can't believe a total stranger was so kind towards me and my family.

When I got to the bedroom, I found Brian at his computer. My happiness from that video vanished when I saw Brian's wide eyes and shocked face. He looked like he had been slapped. "Christina! Fifty/fifty? Is that really what the doctor said to you?"

I felt bad to have given him such a shock. "I'm sorry, Brian. I didn't know you were reading my CaringBridge posts! Yes, he said that. I'm sorry, I just didn't know how to tell you …"

He sat quietly for a minute to gather his thoughts. "Well, there's no fifty/fifty with God," he said. "God is sovereign over this."

YES! Lord, there's no fifty/fifty with you! I have faith you're going to bring all of us through this.

21

ROAD TO RECOVERY

Tuesday, March 31; Thursday, April 2

Balancing the laptop across my thighs, I lay in the cozy hammock on Sean's screened-in porch. It was nice to be in this shady spot, and this morning a lovely breeze was coming through. I opened my computer, hoping to compose a blog post update for my CaringBridge page. I wrote, "Hello Friends! I thought I'd give you a quick update of our COVID journey. It's certainly been very up and down lately......"

I stopped typing when tears began to fall. It had been almost a week since I got home from the hospital, but I was losing confidence I was on the mend. Every day this week was a roller coaster. I had no idea recovering at home would be so hard. I had not vomited since my last trip to the hospital, but my temperature still rose to around 100 degrees at least once a day. My diarrhea had been replaced by constipation, and I still couldn't smell or taste anything. It has been more than a week since my last dose of hydroxychloroquine, but the rash on my back was still very itchy.

Every little activity still left me wheezing and taking shallow breaths, and I worried if the crackles in my lungs were still there. I tried walking with my nieces, but I couldn't go much further than a couple blocks without tiring. Due to the fevers, I had probably taken more Tylenol in these last few weeks than I've taken my entire life. When I wasn't taking my temperature, I kept track of my oxygen levels. Brian bought a pulse oximeter that measures oxygen in the blood, and mine kept hovering around ninety, which was considered a danger zone. I worried every day something would send me back to the hospital. I drank a ton of water and Gatorade. I slept much of the day, and even learned to sleep on my belly because I read an article that said lying face down 'helps improve the condition of your lungs.' I wasn't sure if that was true, but I would try anything.

From inside the house, I could hear the girls in the kitchen eating the breakfast that church members had brought, which was a daily occurrence. I could also hear Brian talking on the phone on yet another work-related conference call. I continuously worry about Brian's health, although he never got nearly as sick as me. He woke up today with a sore throat and has exhibited other symptoms off and on. Thankfully, Sean and the girls have not experienced any symptoms for several days. The girls never complained about anything worse than a few aches and pains, and Sean mostly suffered from some shortness of breath and restless nights. Fortunately, none of us ever developed a cough.

Looking up from the screen, I gazed across Sean's well-manicured lawn, idly watching squirrels and lizards darting through the palm, pine, and oak trees that bordered the yard. I set the laptop aside so I could spray another layer of OFF! on my feet and legs, trying to drive away the persistent no-see-ums that always seemed to fit through the screens. I wished there was some kind of spray to drive away my writer's block.

I'm sure my friends wanted an update on my recovery, but I didn't feel like writing and trying to explain myself to anybody. My phone beeped, and, happy for the interruption, I clicked off the CaringBridge page to pick up my phone.

Sure enough, I got a text "update" from Maxine, the friend who was convinced that I exposed her to the coronavirus at a Bible Study on March 2nd. "Hi Christina, wanted you to know, I'm still not suffering any symptoms from COVID!" I rolled my eyes, glancing at the date on my phone—March 31. I Imagine if she did get COVID-19 now from our last meeting, it would have been the longest incubation period on record!

I guess I just must face the fact that some people might be afraid to be around me, or blame me for giving them COVID, even when I'm fully recovered. It's a fearful and charged climate, and I may face accusations that I acted recklessly by touring around New York City or getting on a plane to Florida. If one more person reminds me to quarantine, I think I'm going to ...

Lord, please help me to deal with insinuations and attacks with no bitterness! You know my heart and intentions, and you have the only opinion I care about. I know I'm incredibly accepted and loved by you! And I'm so blessed that so many people care. I have felt so supported over the past few weeks! So many friends from so many parts of my life have reached out to me in so many ways. It's as if I've been given the chance to attend my own funeral, sitting unseen in the back, while people say nice things about me and remind me of all the good in the world.

I am grateful that my friends in healthcare are still looking after me—happy to give me advice if I have a question about an ache or pain, and they are constantly checking in with me to ask about my lingering symptoms. They reassure me that

I'm on the road to recovery, even though it's not happening as obviously and quickly as I want it to.

I clicked back over to CaringBridge and finished my post. "Brian and I are both feeling the aftershock of dealing with this life-threatening situation. Brian is a prayer warrior, praying loudly and continuously throughout our ordeal, which gives me strength. I have never been the kind who wants to blame God for injustice or cataclysmic events, but I have felt a bit numb spiritually the past few weeks. And yet, I'm convinced that the Holy Spirit is interceding for me. Every day I'm filled with gratitude. I'm so grateful to God for bringing me through this calamity."

I clicked "send" and let out a big sigh.

I looked up as my niece opened the sliding glass door to the porch. "Hey Christina, do you want to go for a walk?" Mae leaned out the door and looked at me hopefully.

"Yes, that's exactly what I need to do," I answered, determined to walk at least one block further than the time before.

I opened up my computer on April 2 and was surprised to receive an email from a lead pastor from Redeemer Presbyterian Church.

Christina, because of COVID, I'm assuming all the short-term mission trips are canceled because of the pandemic, or, at least, they should be. That being the case, and because our church is breaking up into self-governed neighborhood churches, today—April 2—might be the best time to consider transitioning out of your role. The churches can take over from here.

I felt blindsided and went looking for Brian to share this news.

"Brian, I think I just got fired from my job. Wow! An email like that after a whole decade in that job," I complained. "I knew the role was coming to an end, and I know this is probably a good time to let me go because of both the pandemic and our church changing its structure. But—an email? And now, when I've been so sick? I'm not ready to say goodbye to that role. It's almost my identity, in a way. I loved being 'Missions Lady' for all those years."

"I understand," Brian sympathized. "You did a great job with the ministry, and I know you loved it—you were truly called to it."

"I loved going all over the world leading mission trips. It was such an awesome multitasking ministry! It's, like, Christian boot camp for adults—a great way to recalibrate your life as you experience a different culture and see how God works in the world. And we did a *lot* of good. Teammates always came out changed through the experience, the hosts loved us, and we really helped several communities through all those projects we initiated. And you know," I added, breaking into a smile, "I discovered a certain love for Madagascar and South Africa. I'll always feel a call to those countries. I'll miss it."

"But you won't have to miss it, Christina. You can grow your nonprofit and it can still be a blessing. Time to grow and stretch and get creative so you can keep doing international missions, just now through Loving All Nations," Brian encouraged.

Although I felt hurt about the way my missions role had ended, I had to admit that I had been expecting some changes in the role. I said a quick prayer of thanksgiving for what that job had been for me.

Lord, THANK YOU for all the joy and fulfillment and hard lessons that the missions job provided the past decade. Apart from the gift of Brian, I experienced more joy and personal growth from that being in my life than almost anything you've ever brought to me.

Before going to bed that night, I reflected on the past few weeks. Here I was in Central Florida, feeling hopeful and grateful but also chewed up and spat out. I grieved for New York City, which was groaning and gasping as the COVID epicenter of the United States. My heart broke for the world, since the virus was roaring like a lion and causing havoc in every country.

A month ago, I had been lamenting because my life felt impossibly full. I had seen no way to ease my workload or alter my responsibilities that were inked onto every day of my calendar. Now I'd been relieved of my Redeemer job, and I had no idea when anyone might be leading tours around New York City again—even if I regained my strength and stamina to undertake such a physical role. Social engagements and foreign trips were out of the question for the foreseeable future. None of those scribbles in my calendar meant anything at all today.

My life had become unrecognizable within the span of a few weeks!

But, thankfully, I know that our God is sovereign and he is faithful. The Bible assures us that humans will suffer on this earth but also that God is there for us in the midst of our suffering. We're living that reality right now.

22

NEW-BIRTH DAYS

Friday, April 3; Sunday, April 5

"You do the honors, please," I directed Brian, setting the scissors on Sean's dining room table and extending my right arm. "Time to cut off the Hillsborough Hospital ID bracelet! It's been eight days since I left and I'm finally confident that I won't be going back!"

Brian picked up the scissors and snipped the band, holding the long strip aloft in triumph. "You survived! You did it!"

"We *all* survived, and I didn't do anything—God did it."

"Praise the Lord!" Brian and I gave each other a long hug.

The ID bracelet for me symbolized my tie to the virus. I did not want to remove it as long I felt I was just one bad night away from needing to hospital-storm again. Cutting off the bracelet felt like cutting off the power the virus had been holding over me. The hell was truly over, and I was indeed going to live.

Two days later, Brian and I were in the kitchen when my phone buzzed. "Almost there," read the text from Sarah.

Taking Brian by the hand, I led him to the front door. "Sarah and Jeff are coming to drop off food and something *special*," I emphasized. "They're right around the corner—let's meet them outside."

I opened the front door as the familiar red SUV pulled into

the cul-de-sac and sidled up to the curb. Sarah and Jeff jumped out, sprinted to the back of the car, and began pulling bags out of the hatch. Because all five of us were still isolating ourselves, going to a grocery store—or anywhere—was out of the question, and deliveries were still backed up and not a reliable option. Friends who were willing to scour bare shelves to find food for us and then deliver groceries to our front lawn were our lifeline.

"Thanks for the food!" Brian yelled to our masked grocery angels. After the last bag was settled on the lawn next to the curb, Sarah reached into the trunk and pulled out a cake.

She and Jeff began singing, "Happy birthday to you ..." from the curb, and I joined in from our spot by the front door.

They look so funny, standing there on the street by the curb with their big masks on, holding a cake, and singing "Happy Birthday" to Brian while staying twenty feet away.

I looked at Brian, who was smiling at the cul-de-sac serenade. When she finished the song, Sarah yelled, "I'm going to put this on the ground with the rest of the food but hurry up and get it before the ants do! Happy birthday, Brian! We love you!" They waved goodbye, got into the car, and sped away.

As soon as they were gone, we walked to the curb, where Brian picked up several plastic bags while I grabbed the cake. "Groceries and a birthday cake delivered to our curb. Compliments of our best friends."

"It's a birthday we won't forget, will we?" Brian said. "We can share it with Sean and the girls after dinner tonight! It's kind of a birthday for all of us!"

❧

Later in the afternoon I knocked on Janelle's bedroom door.

She opened it, and I shoved a cardboard box into her room dramatically. "Hey, girl! Look what just came from UPS!"

She squealed with delight. "The dresses are here!"

Janelle picked up the box, set it on her bed, broke the tape, and lifted the flap to reveal four full-length formal gowns. She removed the dresses from the box one by one, slid each one out of its plastic sleeve, and draped them across the bed. Soon the comforter was covered with dresses—a luxurious floral, a vibrant red, a classic black, and a metallic bronze. Sequins and embroidered appliqués dripped from the various gowns, and Janelle stopped gazing at them long enough to flash me a wide smile that mirrored my own.

Excited, she tried each dress on and spent several hours creating different hairstyles and makeup palettes to complement each "look." As she modeled in front of me and her full-length mirror, I marveled that I had a niece who was graduating from high school and about to embark on her journey to college.

I was so proud of all she had accomplished in her years of study, and yet devastated she would not be able to fully celebrate those achievements. Thanks to the coronavirus, prom, graduation, senior parties, and honor's banquets had all been canceled. Determined to still find a way to celebrate, Janelle and a small group of her friends planned to hold their own prom outdoors at one of their homes. With stores still closed due to COVID, and her mom deployed out of the country, I wondered how on earth we could find a prom dress. Suddenly I had an idea. I reactivated my Rent the Runway account I had canceled only a week earlier, and together we picked out four dresses so she could choose one to wear to this "home prom."

A home prom was better than nothing, but I grieved for

all the rites of passage my nieces—and all young people—had lost because of this terrible pandemic. But as I looked at Janelle's smiling face, I knew she could come out of this stronger and more resilient than ever if she sought help from God to face these challenges.

As I took pictures of her in each dress, Janelle seemed happy in a way I had not seen since we had fallen ill. I was happy too. Finally, I had found something I could do—even if it would never make up for the miserable trip to New York, or a scary episode of COVID, or a canceled senior prom—so we could have this moment together.

I was filled with hope. Our family will survive COVID, just as Brian and I survived the earlier calamity of the September 11, 2001 attacks. Our lives would never be the same, but we found the strength to carry on. Now I stood on familiar ground, recognizing God's deliverance again, and grateful for God's sustaining grace.

Yet again, I have witnessed the wondrous display of God's providence and mercy firsthand. And I'm so grateful. Lord, YOU are my Rock and my Center. You were with me all the way and brought me onto the other side yet again. Praise to your name, Lord Jesus!

23

RESURRECTED

April 12, Easter Sunday

"C'mon, Christina, you can do it!"

Mae and Janelle were egging me on. With one foot on the pedal, I kicked off from the curb, launching out on my first bike ride in possibly a decade, maybe longer.

"Ughhhhhh! I'm gonna take this seriously slow—you all lead the way and I'll follow."

I wobbled and weaved but gradually got stronger as I aimed to catch up to the girls in front of me. It had been their idea to head outside after we watched a livestream Easter worship service. "Wow, this is fun, y'all!" I yelled as I got more comfortable.

It really is. Maybe I can get into bike riding, since I can't run anymore because of my bad knees.

We rode through back roads and residential streets lined with lovely and interesting Central Florida homes with beautiful oak trees dotting front lawns. After forty-five minutes, the girls pulled over into a park. "Let's take a rest," Mae said, walking her bike to a picnic table. Janelle and I followed.

As we rested and enjoyed the scenery, I voiced words I had been trying to find a way to say for weeks.

"Hey, y'all, I just want to say I'm sorry if I gave the virus to you. That thought has been haunting me ever since we all got sick. I'm so sorry—I must have put you in harm's way somehow. I think we might have gotten it from our train, cab, and boat odyssey when you first got to New York, or maybe I got it before you arrived—maybe while on tour—and passed it on to you."

Janelle stopped me. "Nooooooo. In fact, I'm wondering if *we* gave it to *you*, because I believe we might have gotten sick on the flight up *to* New York." She hesitated for a minute. "I never told you that my throat hurt a little during the entire flight. Like, as soon as we sat down in our seats."

Mae quickly cut her off. "I think we all got it while we were together, although I don't think we'll ever know how. I mean, we could have all caught it on the flight down to Tampa."

Janelle became increasingly serious. "Actually, I'm afraid we would have gone to see our friends right when we came back home because our symptoms were so light. We wouldn't have known we had it. If you and Uncle Brian hadn't come back with us, where you got sick so fast, and we all had to quarantine because *you* had it, we might have exposed our friends to it."

"Wow—what an insight!" I exclaimed. "I had not thought about that." I felt lighter somehow, relieved to know that the girls weren't blaming me for their illness. I had been judging myself more harshly than they were!

"If Brian and I had gotten sick and you had not come to New York City at all, I'm not sure I would have gotten the same hospital care that I did in Florida, and things might not have worked out so great for me. As hard as it was for me to get care here, I know the hospitals in New York were absolutely flooded with cases, so it might have been much worse there.

"And if we had not decided to fly to Tampa to bring you

home, I don't know if we would have left New York. I believe we were meant to come to Florida—it's where we were meant to be treated, and I think God wants us to be here right now, for whatever reason. In fact, I think all of this played out exactly as God planned, which resulted in our health being restored and possibly spared others from being exposed to us."

I brought up another blessing. "And you know what's also nice? We missed the *fear*. We got COVID so early, quickly, and unexpectedly, we didn't have time to develop fear of it. And since we've had it, we don't have anything to be scared of now. We're all antibodied-up! Several of my friends are walking around now *petrified* of getting it. We missed that whole predicament, and I'm so glad we did! We can walk around in confidence—we have freedom from fear!"

"I think we do all the time because of God," added Mae.

Out of the mouths of babes.

As we biked back to their house, I followed behind the girls again. The sky was blue, and it was warm but not oppressively hot. Both girls looked carefree and healthy in their shorts and tank tops, and I watched Mae's long black hair whip up behind her as she pedaled.

I'm following them around on a BIKE in their own community in Florida in April, and we're having a ball. Isn't this topsy-turvy?

Suddenly, I felt a huge sob rising in my chest. The full weight of the past month—all the fear and pain and worry—flashed before my eyes and then was gone, as if it had fallen from my bike basket and tumbled down the street behind us, covered by the dust and gravel we kicked up as we rode forward.

I cannot believe it. It's really over. I'm alive—we're all alive. The girls are as beautiful and healthy as ever. I'm riding a frickin' BIKE.

Look at us—we're the picture of health and contentment and harmony. We MADE IT. Hallelujah! Lord, you did it! You did it! Thank you, thank you!

When we returned home, I joined Brian on the back porch.

"Whatcha doing?" I asked, settling into a lawn chair.

"Oh nothing, just looking through old emails. How was the bike ride?"

"Great," I answered, distracted. Feeling reflective after my bike ride, I felt it was time to tackle a topic I'd secretly been turning over in my mind.

"Brian, I love tour guiding, but I'm hearing it will take a year for tourism to bounce back in New York City. Maybe longer. You've been given the green light to work remotely for the foreseeable future—that means you can work from anywhere! Many of our friends have left the city because of the pandemic. The missions job is ending for me, and our church is livestreaming, like every other church is. The church has been the lynchpin of our community, of our friend base, but now it feels like that role has been diminished. Our life together and individually and what it was made up of seems to be falling—or is being stripped—away.

"We've been down here in Florida quarantining just shy of a month now, and it just feels right to be here. I like the quiet— we can *be* quiet. I was becoming tired of the noise—not just the noise of the city, but noise from all the distractions and running around, while striving for more money to be able to live in one of the most expensive cities in the world. You were right there with me, pushing the limits too. Do you think God might be pushing us to stay in Florida?"

Brian let out a deep breath and said, "I know you love New York City, Christina. You've lived there now, what—twenty-seven years? You love to have fun, and if New York is anything, it's fun. But we are getting older, and the city is changing for us as we age. I'm not sure it's the long-term place for us—not just because we are getting older, but because we could be happy in any environment, including one that's less challenging to live in."

I realized I had been nodding the whole time Brian had been talking. "And I am sure that God will bring us home to him in his perfect timing, but if there is truth to the three-strikes rule, then we've already had two strikes against us. We survived 9/11 and now COVID. I don't want to wait around New York City for strike three! Enough is enough!"

"That's funny—makes me miss the New York Yankees baseball team even more to hear you talk like that!" Brian laughed.

Then he got serious. "Ultimately, it's all about God. Wherever he leads us and whatever he has us do, one thing is for sure—'only what's done for Christ shall last.' We'll keep following him and keep him first, and he'll lead us to whatever future he has in store. It's all good. We can't lose, no matter where we end up!"

EPILOGUE

As a New Yorker, I caught the virus in one of the earliest —and deadliest—waves. After I returned from the hospital and began to recover from this nightmare, I created a document to help others suffering from COVID-19 that I soon shared on social media. As more and more of my friends tested positive, they requested I send them that document. I have written this book as a broader message to help people everywhere know what the disease can look like and how it can feel. I hope my brutal honesty can help anyone fighting this disease or anyone taking care of loved ones who are fighting it. And most importantly, to let them know they are not alone.

I am writing this epilogue at the end of August, more than five months after I exhibited the first symptoms of COVID. My recovery has been far from linear. My energy level and lung capacity are less than half what they used to be. Brian and I have lingering aches and pains, and still make frequent trips to healthcare specialists for mysterious ailments. We have so many different symptoms we've become paranoid about our health. I had a muscle cramp in my calf the other day, and I went into a full-on panic attack that the virus was doing something new. I've heard other survivors express similar fears that this battle may never end.

As a tour guide, I used to walk an average of eight miles per day in Manhattan. But even when I wasn't on tour, I was always on my feet, darting about here and there, preferring to walk over taking the subway. My friends often called me the

Energizer Bunny! No one would call me that now, as I try to get through the day by expending as little energy as possible. I've gained weight as a result of inactivity, which is probably making it even harder for me to walk—a vicious cycle.

Experts in travel are predicting it will be a few years before tourism returns to New York City, especially because there is currently no end in sight to this pandemic. So, for now we will stay in Florida. I will miss the city, my tours, and my activities there. But we will keep the apartment, especially since Brian expects to travel to New York City often for work. I laugh when I remember how little I packed for our "mini-vacation" to Florida! I thought we'd only be gone a few weeks, yet several months later here we are, and I am still living out of that same backpack.

In this book, I have tried to convey how it felt to be living through the early, uncertain days of the novel coronavirus. We had so little to go on. We had daily briefings from the White House, constant updates from Mayor de Blasio and Governor Andrew Cuomo, and guidelines from the CDC. But those guidelines were not always clear, and the messages we received from both the government and healthcare experts were inconsistent and ever-changing.

Facts I referenced here may look inaccurate now, but they are what was known at the time. For example, on March 2nd, the country was reporting that the first COVID-related deaths had occurred on February 28 and March 1 in the Seattle area. We now know that COVID-19 was spreading in the San Francisco Bay area weeks earlier, and other earlier deaths there were later attributed to COVID.

This pandemic was happening so fast that the news

struggled to keep up. We experienced the same uncertainties after 9/11 and watched as official reports were corrected months and even years later. I suspect the same will happen with COVID-19: we will be updating the case counts and death tolls and rewriting the sequence of events for years to come.

New York City was hit incredibly hard by the virus in those early days of spring. Currently, New York is recovering while other parts of the country are seeing skyrocketing rates of illness and death. Florida is now an epicenter of the coronavirus, and many cities resemble New York City in March— closed businesses and empty streets. I left New York thinking I could escape, but instead I moved from one epicenter to another. The virus is everywhere, and there's nowhere left to run.

As I finish writing this book, I am in my hometown of Tallahassee, sitting in a sturdy white rocking chair I bought recently at Lowe's Home Improvement, which I stuffed into our newly leased Kia to transport to the small rental home where we've been living. It's sunny and hot here on the screened-in front porch, and the only sounds I hear are birds chirping in nearby trees.

I take a deep breath as I rock back and forth on the porch, confident that the Lord has led Brian and me here, even as a viral storm rages around us. I have learned many lessons battling COVID, such as the power of prayer and the importance of leaning on the ones God sends to help in times of trouble. He sent people—his emissaries on earth—to help keep me alive. People prayed for me and sent me encouraging words and gave me advice and brought supplies to my door. I will forever be grateful.

The Lord had more plans for my life, and he delivered me from this virus. I was never alone because the Lord was with me. I can't imagine having fought that terrible battle without God.

I'm not sure what the future holds or where life will take us, but this I know: We need the Lord and we need each other. We are better together.

For more information about this book,
visit www.christinaraystanton.com

Made in the USA
Columbia, SC
09 October 2020